LOW BLOOD SUGAR

A Doctor's Guide
to Its Effective Control

LOW BLOOD SUGAR

A Doctor's Guide
to Its Effective Control

J. Frank Hurdle, M.D.

Parker Publishing Company, Inc.
West Nyack, N.Y.

PRINTED IN THE UNITED STATES OF AMERICA
B & P—13-541086-x

TO MY FAMILY

Lee, Claudia, Cathy, Cindy and John,
without whose consideration and forbearance
I couldn't have completed this work.

What This Book Can Do for You

You and I live in a topsy-turvy world. We send men into orbit in outer space, yet we understand little of what goes on in these same men's inner space. Inside their minds, that is. We spend countless millions of dollars in trying to learn what to do about serious illness and caring for people who must be in a hospital, yet we pay scant heed to the man still on his feet—to those of you who may feel pretty good most of the time, but nevertheless spend a lot of days just "feeling rotten," both at work and at home.

How would you like to have a month go by without experiencing a "below normal" day? Even two months or six? Or even a year? How would you like to enjoy robust vigorous health *all the time* for a change? This book will show you just how to accomplish this task.

You don't have to become a superman or have an organ or two transplanted to transform your body into a powerful, well-oiled dynamo of energy and good health. All you need to know is how to effectively control your body's best levels of vital blood sugar. That's what this book is all about—to show you how this is done and why it's necessary for good health.

You've heard much said and may also have read widely concerning the subject of diabetes. It's a fairly common affliction among mankind—there are about 5 or 6 million cases in our country *besides those who are being treated for it!* But here's a fact that is not so generally well known: *For every diabetic there are at least seven or eight people who are suffering the ravages of LOW BLOOD SUGAR!* These seven or eight people may not have low blood sugar all the time, but have it enough of the time to make their physical and mental health suffer because of it. If you're one of these approximately 50 million people in the U.S., this book will help you rejoin the ranks of the healthy again.

Here is another even more interesting fact about blood sugar. Diabetes is a condition in which there is too much sugar floating about in the blood—sugar that isn't being used by the body's cells. The individual body cell, in other words, is unable to use this sugar for energy which it must have in order to function properly. These cells, then, are actually suffering from *not enough sugar*, even though there is too much of it in the blood stream! In low blood sugar (hypoglycemia), though, there is too *little* sugar floating about in the blood stream. The individual cell, and there are trillions of them in your body, has exactly the same problem as in diabetes: *Not enough sugar for the cells to function properly*. How much alike these two conditions are! I'll show you other ways these two conditions are like one another, and what you can do to prevent both of them.

Far too little attention has been given to this condition of low blood sugar (hypoglycemia), and unlike diabetes, for which a patient may take insulin to remedy the condition, you can't "take something" for low blood sugar and expect the condition to be relieved. This book will show you just what you *can* do, however, to correct this vexing condition. And you won't have to make one trip to the local drug store for medication!

Many books have been written about low blood sugar and diabetes. This book is different and more helpful. It explains not only what low blood sugar is, but how to recognize the signs and symptoms of low blood sugar, how to control blood sugar, and what benefits you may expect as a result of this control. Furthermore, this book explains the relationship of low blood sugar to diet, exercise, disease states, and mental health. It even shows how low blood sugar control can help in coping with such serious problems as alcoholism, heart disease, glandular trouble, and nervous disorders.

The key to your good health is in low blood sugar control. Sugar is the body's chief source of energy. Without it, there is no vigor, no will, and no spirit—in short, no satisfactory living. Nature, in her wisdom, has even provided your body chemistry with emergency mechanisms to provide the cells with this vital sugar when the sugar intake falls below the usual level as follows: Proteins taken into your system can be converted to sugar if the need is there. It's highly significant that there is no mechanism in the body for converting sugar into protein in similar crises! Even fats can be metabolized to sugar if necessary. So you may see how important nature feels this vital sugar level is to your well-being.

This book will show you how to take advantage of nature's wisdom.

Perhaps you may recognize the following story: It's mid-morning, and you've dashed into your hectic work day with a scant breakfast, but with plenty of black coffee. A short time later, you begin to feel "empty" in your stomach. This feeling progresses to one of jitteriness, irritability, and near exhaustion. Before noon arrives with its blessed lunch, you're very close to complete physical and mental incapacitation from this syndrome. What you're having is one of the many and variable forms of hypoglycemia, another name for low blood sugar.

If you must wait much beyond your usual lunch time, you may well collapse from sheer "hunger exhaustion." You finally eat—usually to the point of stuffing yourself because of your ravishing hunger. Then you are all right for a couple of hours. At this point the mid-afternoon logginess sets in—you feel stuffed, closed-in, weak, and lacking zip. You're almost useless as far as accomplishing anything is concerned. You have to prod yourself to move. Again, you're having low blood sugar "back-lash," a condition I'll discuss later in the book in detail.

Finally, you arrive home in poor spirits, nerves on edge and feeling bloated. You bark at your family and generally make a bear of yourself around the house. You eat far too much for dinner, get sleepy and have barely enough energy to stretch out on the couch after dinner where you may spend the next two or three hours in a lethargic stupor.

This is but one common set of symptoms associated with low blood sugar. I will go into many others as the discussion continues. The point is, again, you can't take a "miracle drug" for this condition or just dream away the problem. This book will show you what you *can* do, however. If you will only learn to control your blood sugar levels, you can remold your entire health in a very short time, and changes that occur in your mental outlook will literally "make a new person of you." Chronic fatigue, listlessness, lack of energy, depressed personality—will all be things of the past for you.

You can beat the low blood sugar syndrome for an added measure of sparkling good health that can be a revelation to you.

J. Frank Hurdle, M.D.

Table of Contents

11

LOW BLOOD SUGAR

A Doctor's Guide
to Its Effective Control

1

How Low Blood Sugar Control Can Be Your Key to Increased Vitality and Improved Health

What is low blood sugar? Low blood sugar occurs when there is not enough sugar to supply the energy demands of all the cells that make up your body and its organs. Without sugar, or glucose as it's often called, your cells are unable to carry out their vital functions of manufacturing the proteins that make up muscle tissue, or of secreting enzymes and other chemicals that control your heart beat, your breathing, thinking, or of ridding your body of waste materials and poisons.

It is from sugar that body cells get their energy—sugar is the "gasoline" for the engine. Without it, the engine simply won't run.

The control of blood sugar was once thought quite easy: You simply ate sugar, the stomach and intestine absorbed it, and it was either used or stored for future use as the body saw fit. We know now that the control of your body's energy supply is much more complicated than this. What is in the food we eat is not only important, but the *proportion* of various foods and *when* these foods are eaten are equally vital. We also know that physical activity plays an essential role in sugar burn-up—and not only physical acivity, but the very *state of your general health directs blood sugar control.* Also important to sugar control is your body type. It is well known that people who are fat handle their blood sugar much differently from people who are lean.

HOW TO BRING YOUR BLOOD SUGAR INTO HARMONY WITH MENTAL AND PHYSICAL DEMANDS

Your endocrine glands affect blood sugar control. Even your state of mind affects blood sugar control! In fact, it is correct to say that virtually everything you do and everything your body does is geared to the continuous efficient control of blood sugar. You may now see why it's so easy for blood sugar control to get out of hand—and alter your strength, health, and mental outlook so as to run you into the ground. You might be persuaded from this complex problem of the control of blood sugar that there is little that can be done to restore your health and vigor should your blood sugar be low (40 or 50 million of your fellow Americans also have low blood sugar). This is *not* true. It is relatively easy for you to learn how to bring your blood sugar into perfect harmony with the rest of your mental and physical processes. Consider this case.

A Case of Mental Suffering Relieved Through Low Blood Sugar Control

Mrs. S. was a middle-aged, married woman admitted to a mental institution for what was believed to be a "severe reaction to menopause characterized by depression and unwarranted fears." I saw her, as I do all such patients admitted to this mental health center, for her initial physical examination. Mrs. S. was so agitated and nervous that she shook like a leaf on admission. She was hostile, fearful of everyone around her, and complained of symptoms in every system of her body. She couldn't sleep, couldn't eat, and in general was a miserable person to behold.

In the course of examining Mrs. S. medically, and having found her free from any obvious physical disease, it was discovered that she had a marked hypoglycemic reaction during her glucose (sugar) tolerance test. This test is given to observe how the system reacts to a measured amount of ingested sugar over a span of time on an otherwise empty stomach. It's a very useful test in locating both high and low blood sugar, but unfortunately, its use for detecting low blood sugar is not appreciated by many practitioners, who view the test only as a means for the diagnosis of diabetes (high blood sugar).

At any rate, Mrs. S. began to have episodes of fainting with mild convulsions shortly after entering the hospital. Her depression and fearfulness became worse. She did not respond to the usual therapy, and the use of two of the newer drugs for tranquilization only made her worse.

It wasn't until her therapist could be persuaded to stop all her drugs except for a mild sedative at night and to institute a special diet high in protein, high in fats, and low in starches, and to feed this diet in six smaller meals during the day with a bedtime snack, that her fainting and convulsions stopped. She became more calm and rational and began to put on weight. At the same time, she became quite susceptible to psychotherapy and eventually was able to return home, her mental problems under control.

HEALTH PENALTIES INCURRED THROUGH LACK OF BLOOD SUGAR CONTROL

Physicians are often blinded by their own image, and some never seem to learn from experience. For instance, it's a widely held myth in this country that we are the healthiest people on the face of the earth. To some extent this is accurate, but in many ways, it's untrue. Have you seen evidence of doctors' offices containing fewer patients in spite of the fact that medical schools graduate more physicians each year? I haven't. In fact, they're more crowded than ever. Have you seen hospitals with empty beds? I haven't. In fact, I haven't walked into a hospital in the last five years that wasn't either in the process of expansion or had already expanded and planned another in the near future. We're told of the wonderful advances against infectious disease and in the field of preventive health, but people have more infectious disease today than ever—the bugs are just different.

Of course, it's true that we haven't had the Black Plague in

America, nor do we worry much about smallpox anymore, but respiratory infections still attack millions every year and "strep" throat is as rampant as it ever was. Regarding plague and smallpox, with the very serious problem of overpopulation and our relative apathy toward vaccination programs, it's not impossible by any means that either one or both of these pestilences *could* appear again.

The point is this: We are not the healthful Adonises or the immortal Gods and Goddesses that we have been led to believe. If we were, men in their forties wouldn't be dying from acute coronary heart attacks, and there wouldn't be special treatment centers springing up all over the country to treat cancer and strokes.

The Deadly Hidden Menace of Low Blood Sugar

What has all this to do with low blood sugar? Just about everything! Virtually all the major causes of death in the United States today can be linked to the way in which we fail to assist our bodies in handling blood sugar. And this applies to many kinds of accidental deaths, as well as to physical disease! Preposterous? Don't be misled.

Consider heart and blood vessel disease, a leading cause of death among adult males of all ages in our country. The basic lesion in all heart and blood vessel disease is "hardening" of the inside lining of the blood vessels that supply the heart with oxygen and nutrients. The reason for the hardening process has been shown to be deposits of fatty substances in the blood vessel walls. The reason the fatty substances are deposited is that they are in the blood stream in excess amounts. The reason they are in excess is because of overindulgence of improper foods without benefit of physical exercise. *Finally, the reason for overindulgence and lack of exercise is that, initially, improper control of low blood sugar levels triggered the overindulgence and contributed to the lack of energy and will power for proper physical and mental conditioning!*

Thus there is much more to this business of low blood sugar than most of us have been willing to admit.

FAT—THE SILENT KILLER

The problem of obesity is staggering in its proportions in this country. Knowing full well that just being overweight increases the chances of diabetes twelve times, the chances of arthritis eight times, the chances of cancer four times, and the chances of blood vessel disease fifteen times does not seem to deter us from accumulating excess calories and retaining loose, flabby muscles.

There is much we don't know yet about the problem of obesity, but this much we do know: In fat people, sugar tolerance tests are almost always abnormal. Long before diabetes sets in, for example, the sugar tolerance tests are invariably found to indicate *low* blood sugar curves! This, often months or even years before diabetes or another equal disease process makes its appearance. *And at the low blood sugar stage, it is quite possible to reverse the process entirely*—stop the low blood sugar syndrome before it progresses to disease. Moreover, there isn't a physician who hasn't "cured" both diabetes and low blood sugar disorders before they could cause irreversible changes. You can reverse this course yourself!

A Fat Man's Case History

The case of a man I'll call Gus illustrates this point as clearly as any I can recall. Gus was 26 years old when I first saw him in my office. He was five feet, eight inches tall and weighed 272 pounds! He was not solid bone and muscle, but a walking blob of almost pure fat. He came to see me at first because of increasing pain in his shoulders, back and legs. His feet and ankles were swelling such that he couldn't stand to wear ordinary shoes. If he pressed on this ankle swelling he noticed it left a deep indentation in his skin for several minutes, the sign of a failing heart. He was short of breath so much of the time that he couldn't walk a half block before he felt as though he were going to pass out from sheer exhaustion and lack of oxygen. He also noticed increasing dizziness and inability to rest comfortably when he lay flat in bed.

In taking Gus's history, I learned he was perfectly well until only five years ago when he began to put on weight. He didn't think much about it because, as he stated it, "All my people were big." He also reluctantly recalled that none of these "big" people had lived beyond their fifth decade!

Gus seemed to crave sweets and starchy foods and figured "his body needed it," so he gave it plenty. Things got out of hand. The more he ate, the more he craved. He worked in a job which put considerable pressure on him, and this, too, induced him to eat as a means to combat the "nervous feeling" this pressure caused. He had tried many diets, doctors, specialists, and so on without lasting results. His increasing discomfort and long list of symptoms brought him to my office, not because of any reputation of mine, but because he was desperate and in sheer agony.

I told Gus that before I'd take his case or even try to deal with any of his numerous symptoms, he'd have to promise to let me examine him carefully with certain tests and agree to follow subsequent advice to the letter. He was willing to do anything if he could get relief from his widespread arthritis, fatigue, and shortness of breath.

Gus's sugar tolerance test surprised me. I felt certain he had diabetes, as well as heart failure and arthritis. Instead, his sugar tolerance curve indicated both a diabetic curve at the start *and a low sugar curve* at the end! How could this be? Something wrong with the laboratory results, maybe? Decidedly not. A repeat test a few days later demonstrated this same "opposite" reaction. The answer wasn't as difficult as it appeared. Gus's sugar curve just showed that not only was his body unable to handle sugar once it reached his bloodstream (the diabetic situation), but once his sugar levels reached an unusually high concentration, his body's response to it was overwhelming and his sugar levels were driven down to abnormally low levels where they persisted until the next meal or snack (the hypoglycemic, or low blood sugar situation).

When Gus lost 80 pounds of his flab, regulated his diet, and worked a regular course of graduated exercise into his daily routine, he proceeded to get well. Within a year, he regained his wind, his ankle swelling stopped, and his sugar tolerance curve returned to entirely normal levels. Another six months and 30 pounds of weight loss later saw his arthritic pains cease altogether.

Gus was on the verge of developing full blown diabetes. He demonstrated the typical low blood sugar syndrome that often precedes this disease and which is the cause of the sweets and starch overindulgence that fully seven diabetics in ten show before they develop their disease. He headed his trouble off without doing a thing you can't also do. And with a good deal less strain and pain, since I'm betting you haven't let things get quite as far out of hand as Gus had!

HOW BLOOD SUGAR CONTROLS VITAL LIFE PROCESSES

To understand how you can control low blood sugar and enjoy better health as a result is to understand how blood sugar enters into your vital life processes, what factors enter into its regulation, and the things you can do to bring blood sugar into harmony with the rest of your body functions.

Where does the body's supply of blood sugar come from? A reasonable first question. Your body gets its sugar either in pure form or from starchy foods. Table sugar, the white crystalline substance you put in your morning coffee and use to sweeten your cereal, is pure, unadulterated glucose. It comes from the sugar beet or from sugar cane grown in the tropics. You might say table sugar is pure biologic energy, just as gasoline is pure engine energy for your car.

Starch foods supply sugar in high amounts. The sugar in starchy foods isn't pure like table sugar, but is formed in the body by a relatively simple breakdown of a class of chemicals called carbohydrates, found in foods like spaghetti, potatoes, bread, and pastries, to list a few. In addition to carbohydrates, proteins and fats constitute the two other major chemicals in the food you eat. Following digestion, all foods yield one or more of these three general types of chemicals. All are needed by your body to survive. In addition, vitamins, minerals, enzymes and roughage are also needed, but these chemicals are not directly utilized in your body's nutrition. They merely help in the breakdown and storage of the three main food chemicals.

When You Feel the Need for "Quick Energy"

Let's trace what happens when, for instance, you feel the need for some "quick energy" and eat a teaspoon or two of table sugar to supply it. The sugar reaches your stomach where, because of its purity and lack of need to be further digested, it's absorbed directly into your bloodstream. Immediately, your circulation carries the sugar to virtually every cell in your body. This happens in a matter of seconds! The sugar is absorbed by the body cells in need of it and the sugar is "burned" inside the cell to carbon dioxide (the same carbon dioxide that we exhale as we breathe), and to water. In this process of "burning," the cell has received energy which it uses in thousands of ways in performing its amazing functions. In the brain, much of this energy is used by cells in thinking—as you read this page, your heart cells are using sugar for energy to contract—become smaller—in the process of pumping blood throughout your system. As you read this page, your blood cells are using energy in high quantities so that your blood flow will keep up the steady pace necessary to keep you alive.

But besides being "burned" by the cells, this bit of sugar you've taken in has also started a number of other reactions in your body. As it circulated through your pancreas gland, it stimulated the cells of this organ to secrete insulin, without which your cells could not "burn" the sugar presented to them. The insulin-secreting pancreas gland is one of your body's "double organs." That is, it not only delivers chemicals to your digestive tract that help digest starches and proteins, but it is also one of the endocrine glands—the glands of your body that deliver chemicals directly into the bloodstream and control the very life functions without which none of us could survive. Nature has seen fit in her wisdom to include this process of sugar burning in her vital processes. And she has given this function prime consideration in more ways than one, as we shall soon see.

Glandular Reactions to Sugar

As the sugar circulates through your pituitary gland, another endocrine gland located at the base of your brain, this gland is stimulated to deliver a chemical into your bloodstream that slows down the insulin secreted from your pancreas so that the pancreas will not be tempted to oversupply insulin to burn the sugar. At the same time, another chemical from the pituitary gland is released that influences yet a third endocrine gland, the adrenal gland, to act to stimulate your liver to release some of its stored sugar for the insulin to burn as a safety feature to insure that the insulin will have "enough to work on" and not get overactive.

As a matter of fact, the far-reaching influence of the pituitary gland over all the other endocrine glands in your body has earned it the title of "the body's master gland," and the name is well deserved. There is not a function that occurs inside your body that the pituitary gland is not in direct or indirect control of. Is it not significant that nature has placed sugar control in the lap not only of the master endocrine gland, but also the adrenal, the pancreas, and to a lesser extent, the thyroid gland?

Sugar control is indeed the essence of the healthy cell in virtually every gland, every muscle, and every nerve fiber in your body. *Learning to control sugar levels in your body is the key to full health, vigor and mental development.* You can learn this control easily. It isn't too late to start even if you aren't in the "prime" of life, and even if you may be in poor physical shape now.

HOW VITAL BLOOD SUGAR IS STORED IN LIVER

Previously, I mentioned the liver as the storage depot of sugar. Next to the brain, the liver stands out as the body's most versatile organ. Although it is not one of the endocrine glands, the liver takes care of 20 or more different functions of your body's metabolism. When this organ gets out of whack, you can expect nothing but trouble!

Among other substances, the liver stores sugar when it's not immediately needed by your body's cells. This it does by combining several molecules (single units) of sugar together to form a compound called *glycogen*. In this form, the sugar is stored inside the liver cells until the body calls for a supply. When it does, the glycogen is "split" into separate sugar units again and rushed directly to the bloodstream.

The liver has a remarkable capacity to recuperate when it's damaged. This is primarily because it's so large, occupying the entire right upper one third of your abdomen. Because of its large size and because of the fact that its cells perform so many different functions, liver cells themselves use a tremendous quantity of sugar. So when something goes wrong with the sugar levels, liver cells are unable to do many of their jobs. For instance, they may lose their ability to break down fats and manufacture proteins, the building blocks of all cells. You can see what a vicious circle of disease starts when blood sugar levels go astray!

The Case of an Alcoholic's Liver

I recall a case of a middle-aged man who, because he had been a heavy drinker for 20 years, had rather pronounced damage of the liver when he came to my office. He had finally become a staunch member of alcoholics anonymous and climbed on the wagon permanently. I encouraged him, and he was able to follow through, to get his weight down and increase his carbohydrate intake at the same time. This sounds as though it might be impossible, but I assure you it isn't, as we'll see later. Under this regime and without drugs of any sort, his liver function returned to the point where his metabolism was within normal limits. He prevented an early death for himself by simply taking advantage of nature's built-in capacity for recovery, using blood sugar control as the basis for his own therapy.

HOW RESISTANCE TO DISEASE IS BOLSTERED BY PROPER BLOOD SUGAR LEVELS

Even your body's ability to resist infection depends on the integrity of blood sugar controls.

The body's resistance to viral and bacterial infection is primarily a function of the lymphatic system. These lymph glands, which are located throughout your body, and the blood cells that are developed in them and from your bone marrow, are your first line of defense when infection strikes.

When a germ invades your organism, its character and structure are determined by the lymph structures. The way this is done is very much like making a key that fits a certain lock, as follows: The germ itself is of a certain protein structure with dents and bumps on its tiny surface. The cells of the lymph and blood form a blueprint of these dents and bumps as they come into contact with the invading germ. Immediately these cells start to manufacture proteins that exactly fit the holes and grooves on these germs, thereby rendering them harmless. These neutralizing proteins are produced in tremendous amounts and engulf the bacteria as they begin their invasion, blocking them or neutralizing them so they cannot attack the body cells against which they're active.

This manufacture of tremendous amounts of protein blocking agents, called antibodies, takes fantastic amounts of energy in the cells that are making them. And what happens if there aren't enough reserves of sugar? Not enough antibodies are made, and the germs take over.

This is why certain thin, pale, asthenic individuals who are weakly constituted fall prey to so many bugs that are "going around" and are sick with one thing or another most of the time. Their cells just don't have the energy available to them to build their resistance to such germs. Once reconstituted, such individuals are fully capable of being healthful, vigorous individuals again. All they need is a more carefully regulated blood sugar supply.

A Case History of Chronic Fatigue

The case of Jane W. is an example of what I mean. Jane was 30 years old when I first saw her in my office. She was about 30 pounds underweight, pale, and wan. She was nervous, weepy and blamed all her troubles on her poor husband, a vigorous muscular man who looked ten years younger than Jane though both were the same age.

She complained of chronic fatigue, being run-down all the time, and had a list of illnesses and symptoms covering a full

page on the record sheet. Careful questioning revealed that Jane
was the weakling of the family—the "runt" of several brothers
and sisters that were vigorous, athletic people. She was pampered
and babied through her childhood, and had been treated somewhat like a fragile flower. I honestly don't think Jane ever knew
what good nutrition was, since she was allowed to eat or not as
she pleased and never got much of a chance to burn off any
energy in playing like others her age. She was a classic example
of a ninety pound weakling.

A short course of hospitalization revealed that no real disease
was behind Jane's sorry physical state. Her blood sugar curve,
however, was quite revealing. It showed that her levels of available sugar were far below normal on an empty stomach, and
that on drinking a measured amount of sugar water and testing
her blood levels, her sugar was burned so rapidly that it fell
very shortly to levels even lower than her below normal fasting
levels! So much, in fact, did her sugar level fall that she went
into a low sugar shock-like state as a direct result of the test!

Jane, fortunately, had had quite enough of her dilemma. She
was willing to do most anything to feel well again. Within three
months, on a special diet and graduated exercises at home, she
gained 15 pounds, and a change occurred in her mental outlook
that was a wonder to behold. Instead of the depressed, weepy,
blame-it-all-on-someone-else-attitude, she became assertive, self-
reliant, and a real wife to her husband. She no longer retreated
from making friends and attending social functions, and soon
became not only able to keep up with her vigorous husband, but
actually acquired more stamina than even he could match!

Not only that, but Jane hasn't had a cold, the flu, or any other
infection, viral or bacterial, since this change. This is proof positive that resistance does, indeed, depend not only on blood
sugar control, but on your state of mind as well.

HOW YOUR MIND DEPENDS ON PROPER BLOOD SUGAR

Why is there reference to the state of mind and your blood
sugar levels? Sound like hocus-pocus? At first, yes, but actually, it
is far from it!

For many years, scientists were unaware of the many functions of the human brain. They knew, or were reasonably certain, that the brain was the seat of the mind, and that it served a kind of "switch-board" function as far as the nerves were concerned. Little did they suspect that the brain was infinitely more versatile than they'd ever dreamed. For example, it's known that the brain itself secretes certain chemicals like the endocrine glands do. Some of these chemicals go directly into the bloodstream where they are carried to their "target organs," others are secreted directly into the pituitary, the master endocrine gland we've already talked about. It is no wonder nature located the pituitary at the brain's base and provided nerve circuits directly from it to various brain centers!

This discovery, not too many years ago, answered a host of unexplained questions. The things psychiatrists were saying had their source in the mind now began to make much more sense to the average doctor who, before this time, had a difficult time trying to figure how, for instance, the mind could possibly affect the function of an endocrine gland or other organ located far away in the body. The new knowledge also filled in many gaps about how the mind could be affected by changes in the body. There was now a complete circuit to explain this vague phenomenon. For example: Suppose you are suddenly startled or frightened—stimulated, in other words, by a strong emotion. The emotion centers in the brain, in turn, stimulate the pituitary (either through direct nerve connections, or by chemicals, or both) to secrete less of its dampening effect on insulin. The "released" insulin burns the sugar necessary for the immediate energy needed for the situation causing the fright. The pituitary also stimulates the adrenal glands to secrete adrenalin which keys up your muscles and prepares you for defense, and to prod your liver to break down its glycogen supply for the increased sugar your body will need for its increased energy. Then the fright passes. The situation is taken care of in one way or another, and the emotional situation is gone. The pituitary is no longer stimulated, and your other organs resume their normal state. What harmony of teamwork! What a grand system of checks and balances nature works in the human organism!

In Jane W.'s case previously described, one can imagine how her poor mental attitude dampened her emotional controls, thence affected her pituitary, thence, her endocrine gland function. This is only a single example of how mind and body function as a whole—as an integrated and intimately bound-up unit. It also shows how blood sugar control is absolutely *vital* to this teamwork between mind and body.

WHY MUSCLES NEED SUGAR

We now arrive at a consideration of muscle tissue and its connection with blood sugar control.

Muscle tissue comprises most of the total mass or weight of your body. The prime function of muscles is to perform work. Mostly, this work is against the force of gravity which acts to pull you toward the earth's surface. This pull must be overcome at all times if we are to remain in an upright position. The only time, in fact, that this gravitational force isn't being overcome is when we are flat in bed or on the ground. Think of the energy required of muscle cells just in keeping us standing!

Besides your skeletal muscles, which include all the muscles over which you have direct control, your entire digestive apparatus is a muscular tube, constantly in motion in the process of digestion and elimination of waste. In addition, your heart is nothing more than a tremendously strong muscular pump that pushes gallons of blood through your blood vessels every day of the year without rest of any kind, except for the split-instant after the second of the two heart sounds! Think of it! A small organ like the heart constantly doing the work of a heavy duty engine without being turned off even once!

Muscle Waste Products Must Be Eliminated

But muscle tissue, particularly those we have voluntary control over, is peculiar in that if the wastes that accumulate in its cells aren't promptly removed, the efficiency of the muscle degenerates. And no matter how much energy a muscle cell has available to it, if the waste products have been allowed to pile up, it can't be anything but totally inefficient. This means that muscles must have an efficient waste removal system if they're to work properly. The one thing that removes muscle cell waste is *exercise*.

The Flabby Muscle Syndrome Case History

I recently talked to a former college football player who had become a high-powered insurance executive. He complained that he did his work all right, but was completely exhausted when he got home, and thus had absolutely no energy to involve himself with his family. In the course of our discussion, I reminded him that not only had he gained about 35 pounds since his college football days, but he had done nothing to keep his muscles in shape since he graduated into the business world. When he began a systematized daily routine of exercise, his fatigue and excess weight disappeared completely. He told me later that he'd never felt so good, had energy and zip to spare, and fatigue never bothered him since he'd started his exercising.

This man's story is well worth remembering because millions of Americans suffer from the flabby muscle syndrome. And the reason for it is that their sugar levels suffer because of their inability to utilize effectively their energy stores. Their sugar is stored as glycogen, then when the storage bins are full, their sugar is turned to fat and flab. As a consequence, their circulating sugar is below normal, and they feel loggy and listless most of the time.

Remember, too, that although you don't have direct control over your involuntary muscles, like your heart or digestive tract, these muscles are no different in their response to exercise from voluntary muscles. Every time you exercise your abdominal muscles, for example, you tone up the muscles of your intestine as well. By the same token, exercise of all kinds tones up the heart muscle. Athletes have smaller, more efficient hearts, even though their hearts do more work than non-athletic hearts. This is why an athlete's heart has a decidedly slower pulse rate, often 20–30 beats a minute slower than an average non-athlete's heart. Their hearts are just that much more efficient because of the exercise their bodies get.

Blood Vessel Muscles Need Conditioning

The outermost lining of your blood vessels, especially the arteries that carry blood to your muscles and organs, are made of muscle. When this muscular coat stiffens up for any reason, high blood pressure is the result. High blood pressure causes damage to internal organs and to the heart, and is a major cause of strokes. Isn't it sensible to keep the muscular coats of these arteries in tone so that such trouble may be prevented? Of course it is! And the way to do this is, again, through exercise. Even small arteries have even smaller channels in them which carry blood to the artery wall—the muscular coating that surrounds them. If, by proper dieting and exercise, the waste from these artery muscles is carried away efficiently, and if the blood sugar levels are kept at optimal levels, you stand an excellent chance of never having to worry about high blood pressure!

The discussion regarding muscles wouldn't be complete without mention of another group of muscles so small that most people don't consider them muscles at all, but, as anyone with asthma or emphysema can tell you when their lungs go into spasm, they do, indeed, exist. I'm speaking of the thin muscular coating around the millions of little air sacs in your lungs. These muscles, too, require constantly controlled blood sugar levels and elimination of waste to perform at top efficiency. Control of exercise, diet and blood sugar levels helps insure that they do their job properly.

SUMMARY

1. The control of blood sugar levels is the key to every facet of your good health. Blood sugar is the sole source of energy to the cells that make up every part of your organism.
2. The endocrine glands are the first line of blood sugar control. Since these glands also control virtually every vital function of your body and mind, their top efficiency is necessary to achieve blood sugar control.
3. Your brain, in turn, exerts control of these endocrine glands. The cells of your mind located in the brain must have proper

levels of blood sugar to properly control the glands and to enable you to think and work efficiently. You must keep both body and mind in peak condition, therefore, if you are to be an efficient organism.

4. Most of the common diseases afflicting mankind today are directly or indirectly linked to low blood sugar levels. These are:

   Heart disease and high blood pressure.
   Obesity, arthritis and diabetes.
   Gall bladder disease, digestive disorders, and cirrhosis of the liver.
   Mental disorders, infections, and a good proportion of accidents and injuries.

5. Since the prevention of low blood sugar and all its complications depends on the smooth working of the entire body-mind complex, you must bring these vital functions under optimal control and keep them that way.

6. As a part of a program to achieve blood sugar control, the following must become part of your daily concern:

   Proper diet.
   Proper exercise.
   Proper sleeping and breathing habits.
   Proper health precautions.
   Proper mental attitudes.
   Proper work and recreational programs.

2

How to Recognize Low Blood Sugar Symptoms

How many times have you said to yourself, ". . . If I'd only known it was happening, I could have prevented it" or, "If someone had only told me. . . ."? All of us have reason for making such statements. This only proves we're human. In the helter-skelter of everyday living, we tend to ignore things that to us seem simple and clear enough, but to somebody else, particularly if he's feeling poorly, may not be clear at all. How many times I've heard patients say, "I wish someone had explained all this to me before"!

Low blood sugar in its early stages produces a variety of signs and symptoms. These sympoms are here discussed so that you may better recognize them and head them off before they start a series of events leading to poor health.

You may instantly recognize some of these symptoms. Others may have seemed to you merely "part of life that must be endured." Now you can do away with them forever. You'll recall earlier I made the statement that virtually *every facet of your health* is hinged on the proper control of blood sugar. This applies to the "little aggravations" that affect your physical well-being, as well as to the major diseases that may well result from neglect of these small, often transient disorders. The next chapter will deal with corrective diet and nutrition.

HOW TO AVOID THE LOW BLOOD SUGAR "BLUES"

1. Fatigue

Cases of chronic fatigue probably number in the tens of millions in this country every day. Almost everyone has had the experience of feeling exhausted long before his day's work is done. But when the symptom of fatigue becomes a habit, you're on the way to a chain reaction that can only spell trouble. When you feel "bushed," even after adequate rest, ask yourself this question: *"Do I have any other signs of disease?"* If the answer is *"no,"* suspect low blood sugar as the most likely culprit.

Two Kinds of Fatigue

Remember that there are generally two kinds of fatigue: (1) The natural pleasant fatigue that results from vigorous healthful exercise with almost any kind of physical activity. This fatigue is restful and natural; it's good for you. Learn to savor it, since it reflects good balance in your daily routine. (2) The other kind of fatigue is the dragged-out, raw-edged, nervous fatigue. Learn to recognize this latter fatigue as the sign of poor blood sugar control and as a warning that something must be done.

Of course, fatigue of this second type also occurs with states of disease. But remember that *there are always other symptoms that go along with the disease besides fatigue.* If, with fatigue, you notice shortness of breath, chest pain and stomach distress, it follows that medical help should be consulted, and the necessary things done to find out what is causing this *group* of symptoms of ill health. But fatigue by itself calls for action on *your* part. And it can be eradicated by proper attention to the low blood sugar which causes it.

2. Headache

Of physical symptoms complained of most by all the people in the United States, the headache heads the list. For many reasons, the symptom of headache often strikes fear into the heart of the person who has it. The first reason is that it has become an automatic connection in far too many people that headache and brain tumor are practically synonymous. This is a myth and a complete fairy tale. Like all such fantasies, this myth contains a small grain of truth in that, having progressed far enough, most brain tumors can produce a headache.

Such a headache is usually *the last symptom* that a brain tumor causes, there being a host of other well-recognized signs occurring before headache starts. The same can be said of the other fear-causing kind of headache: That produced by something drastically wrong with the blood vessels within the head, often called a stroke or vascular accident.

As a matter of fact, the chances of headache being caused by one of these two serious disorders is very small indeed. On the other hand, the chances of headache being caused directly or indirectly by blood sugar disorders is extremely high!

The most common cause for headache is tension! Tension is caused by a high level of nervous anxiety about almost anything. Such accumulation of nervous tension can be a by-product of low blood sugar levels! Another common kind of headache is the so-called migraine type of headache. This variety of head pain is seen more often in women than in men, though it can occur in either sex, and tends to appear in the female side of a person's family history. That is, your mother, grandmother, aunt, or all three may have had this disorder at one time or another in their lives. This migraine type headache is an effect of nervous tension upon the blood vessels inside the head, and, like the tension headache, is strictly a product of an inefficient escape valve for excess and unusual nervous stress.

Again, if you are in control of your blood sugar, thence your nervous system, migraine headaches become conspicuous by their absence!

You can sort out serious headaches from those caused by low blood sugar in the following manner: If you have headaches when you first awake in the morning; that cause any disturbance of your eyesight (double images, rainbow colors around electric lights, blindness); or that are associated with any trouble with the proper coordination of your fingers, hands, arms, legs, or with a state of unconsciousness (fainting or convulsions), medical advice should *always* be sought. Otherwise, you may be assured that your headache relief is in the province of control of blood sugar levels.

3. Insomnia and Nightmares

Sometimes you go to bed, tired and worn out, feeling as if you could drop in your tracks and probably fall asleep in a chair if necessary. You hit the bed, but try as you will, sleep doesn't come. You toss and turn, count sheep, talk to yourself, drink a glass of fizzy alkalizer, but all to no avail. You have insomnia. Finally, when sleep does come, after pacing the floor, you wake up with a jolt, having had a revolting dream—a nightmare.

The reason for insomnia and nightmares is that you went to bed physically ready for sleep but with a problem on your mind. The problem caused indecision—a conflict arose and "bugged" you so much you couldn't sleep, or if you did, the conflict pops up again in your dreams. You *can* control this indirect symptom of poor blood sugar regulation.

In fact, all three parts of what I've called the low blood sugar blues are definitely under your control. The question whether the fatigue, headache and insomnia with nightmares *caused* altered metabolism and low blood sugar, or whether altered metabolism with low blood sugar *causes* the fatigue, headache or insomnia with nightmares condition really isn't too important. It's no more important than trying to answer the question whether the chicken came before the egg or the reverse. The point that *is* important is: Your altered state of mind and body *do exist,* and working at cure from either end of the scale will produce results. From a chicken you can get an egg, and from an egg you can get a chicken.

Let's consider *fatigue.* The kind of fatigue that sets in far too soon in the day to be physically caused—the kind that leaves you feeling like you've been dragged through a wringer—the kind you may wake up with in the morning. Fatigue comes on as a result of anything that's *depressing* to you. Something that's getting you down. Being constantly mad and hostile at something or somebody can induce it. It's a well-known fact that the best way to work off anger and hostility is to release all the pent-up "madness" from its walled off interior—get rid of it by making a vent through which it can escape. How is this done? The very act of physical conditioning, which we'll soon see as one of the prime necessities in maintaining proper blood sugar levels, is one of the best methods.

Physical conditioning has at least two effects on fatigue. The first is that physical exercise calls on the endocrine system, the set of glands we learned about in the first section that control your body's vital functions, to stimulate blood circulation in the brain. This carries away accumulated waste products of cell metabolism and delivers vital blood sugar to the cells that depend absolutely on a constant supply of this vital substance. The second effect is that, as we've also learned, muscles in good tone have an effect on brain cells that "tones" them as well—the metabolism inside the brain cells is stimulated and speeded up, restoring the vigor of the cells that are responsible for bright, alert minds.

The same can be said for the *common headache*. Whatever the cause for the nervous tension, followed by stiffening and pain in the neck muscles, scalp, and finally the forehead, relief of pain follows the toning up of stiff neck muscles or any other muscles of your body, and the restoration of proper diet furnishes enough sugar for those fatigued muscle cells so that they no longer get stiff and sore!

As for *insomnia with nightmares,* there is nothing better for sleepless nights than 15–20 minutes of well-controlled *physically* fatiguing exercise coupled with maintenance of proper levels of blood sugar throughout the day.

Finally, a direct attack on the emotional and mental problems that bring symptoms of low blood sugar blues to the fore depends on your ability to focus a few of the marvelous powers that reside in your mind, but largely go begging from not being used! Your powers of mind depend on constant attention to blood sugar levels for their efficient function.

HOW TO COPE WITH THE "JITTERS": LOW BLOOD SUGAR AT ITS WORST

An Aggravated Case History

The last middle-aged man I saw with shakiness was convinced he had Parkinson's Disease, a neuro-muscular condition caused by damage to some of the deep centers of the brain. He had resigned himself to live the life of a cripple and to expect an early death. The potent drugs he'd been given to stop his shaking hands, arms and legs had dried up his mucous membranes so thoroughly that he could hardly swallow, and had constipated him so badly that he'd become completely dependent on laxatives. In addition, this unfortunate man had lost 45 pounds of weight, pounds he couldn't afford to lose.

In talking with him, I learned that his shakes and jittery nerves started about a year ago, just after he'd been promoted to a responsible position in the company in which he worked long and hard hours to reach the top. He'd been overwhelmed by all this responsibility and had taken to drinking huge quantities of coffee during the day and more liquor than he should have at night. The shakes came on in full force. He lost more and more time at work, and finally took a leave of absence in hopes of finding solace and cure. Unfortunately, running away from his problems only made things worse.

The Low Blood Sugar Culprit

When I talked him into going to the hospital for a few days of rest and tests, I noticed his shaking improved materially after only two days of freedom from worry and stress and the benefit of mild sedation at night. The next day, his blood sugar test came back. His curve looked like a mountain ski slope! His sugar level before eating was on the lower side of normal, certainly nothing to be excited about, but at two hours following his drinking of the measured sugar solution, his sugar level was 15 per cent below the fasting (before meal) level, and at four hours fell to 50 per cent below the fasting level! During the test his shakes flared in all their glory but responded promptly to glucagon, a drug used to stimulate the liver to release some of its reserve sugar deposits. Once it became obvious that this man suffered from the low blood sugar jitters, the institution of a correct diet, physical conditioning, and *decreased* coffee and alcohol relieved him of shakes forever. Later, he was able to face his responsibilities without fear and trepidation and is to this day a successful and highly respected manager in his company.

Side-Effects to Watch

With these jitters, may also come an unexplained weakness: A real loss of physical strength. The loss of strength can occur in people with fairly good muscle tone, but seems decidedly worse in people with loose, flabby muscles. Strength loss is most pronounced following a cup or two of black coffee on an empty stomach, or following the use of too much alcohol before mealtime. Adding cream or sugar to coffee or eating right away after a few drinks may alleviate the low blood sugar weakness, but usually, if you'll notice carefully the next time, there is that prolonged feeling of half-nausea, half-giddiness that may persist for several hours. Low blood sugar levels do leave their mark!

WHEN THE CHEST POUNDS AND THE HEAD REELS

Heart or Low Blood Sugar Trouble?

There are few things more freightening than to honestly believe you're having a heart attack. Such was the stark terror on the face of a young lady in her 30's whom I saw in the emergency room of a hospital not long ago. It seems that she'd been a frail and weak person most of her life, but had never had anything seriously wrong with her health—so she thought. She was subject to palpitations and episodes of dizziness. This particular night, she had been to a social gathering with friends and had eaten many of those little pieces of foreign-made bread filled with rich sea-food, candy, and a glass or two of sherry wine. Toward the end of the evening, our freightened lady was taken with a sudden burst of "heart pounding," the likes of which she couldn't remember in the past. Her pulse was wild and her heart, to use her own words, was "fluttering and turning flip-flops" inside her chest cavity. She was seized with panic. After all, wasn't she subject to "heart trouble" anyway? Wasn't she weak and liable to have a catastrophe any day?

When I began to examine her, I noticed something about her eyes. They seemed to be jerking from side to side, especially when she tried to glance sideways. I asked her to sit up. She did, and received another horrible shock when the objects in the examining room, including, she gasped, her doctor, began to spin around in crazy circles. Shortly after this, she vomited, then felt much better.

I had the laboratory draw a small sample of blood from my patient so that the lab technician could perform a screening blood sugar level. This is a quick, immediately available trick with a chemically impregnated piece of tape that gives the general range of the blood sugar. It isn't as accurate as the sugar tolerance test or the sugar level test done on an empty stomach over four to five hours time, but it is very helpful for immediately estimating a situation. The range of this lady's blood sugar proved to be less than 50 mgm. per cent—a level 25 mgm. per cent below what it should have been with her stomach completely empty!

Over a period of time, this woman was able to control her blood sugar through a concerted effort at diet and exercise. As time went on, she changed in many ways. She emerged from her cocoon of fears, embarrassments, and delusions of all kinds of physical ailments, including the one centered around her heart. Subsequently, she married, had a family, and became literally a new woman. To my knowledge, she has never had palpitation, heart flutters or vertigo (dizziness that seems to make the objects in the surroundings spin), since this episode.

THE "BLAHS"—WHAT TO DO ABOUT THEM

The "blahs" are common to low blood sugar states. "Blahs" occur when you feel completely and disagreeably listless, have no drive or ambition to do anything, and what's more, you just don't care about anything. "Blahs" aren't usually helped much by taking any of the many kinds of fizzy drinks offered on today's market. The "blahs" can be *completely eradicated by correcting low blood sugar,* as you will be guided in this book.

What causes you to have the "blahs"? Suffocation of your alert mechanism, to say it simply. In your brain there is a special area deep within its substance that is concerned with the control of your alert or awake state of mind. At night when you go to bed, the alert center is "turned off" and sleep follows. In the morning, this center is "turned back on" again, and you are awake, ready to take on the day's problems. If, for some reason, the center is partly or completely slowed up during the day, you have the "blahs."

The onset of the "blahs" may lead you to think you may be coming down with the flu or some other such malady. Moreover, if you don't do something about the "blahs," you may, in fact, actually come down with a cold or some other "bug"! The reason for this is that during the "blahs" your resistance and immunity systems don't function properly—if the "blahs" are left to their own design, your health can suffer.

The other trouble with the "blahs" is that during this lowered efficiency state, none of the rest of your usually dynamically functioning brain is able to function very well either. You feel sluggish and unable to carry through with ideas or plans that require thought. And you can't push yourself to do what you know needs doing. As your low blood sugar again attains proper levels, "blahs" become a thing of the past, and you can be the vital human being you should be again and start accomplishing what you want without the slightest effort.

With correction of your "blahs," you can once again start to concentrate on the tasks at hand. As we shall see later, concentration is the mental key to creative productivity. With the "blahs," you simply can't produce.

HOW TO COMBAT THE STUFFED-UP SYNDROME

We Americans are an affluent people, and our eating habits show it. I've talked to literally hundreds of people over the years who think nothing of stuffing themselves so tightly at dinner time, that they become stupefied and spend the rest of the evening dozing or sleeping in a chair or couch. It's no wonder they can't sleep the rest of the night or that their health seems to suffer.

What happens at "stuffing time" is simple, when you look at it closely. The reason for all the food cramming is that we come home *with the low blood sugar state already well started.* Overeating is giving in to the terrific hunger pangs in your stomach. And when your body is crying for food, you always overdo. You eat like a starved animal and end the gluttonous process by forcing down a rich dessert, even though you can't possibly hold "another bite." Why? Why indulge this almost overwhelming drive to eat yourself into the grave? *Because low blood sugar levels will not be put off!*

Low blood sugar levels must be *prevented* if the stuffed-up syndrome plagues you. Here's what happens if you don't watch yourself:

1. Arrive at the dinner table starved, eat until stuffed. Blood sugar, extremely low before mealtime, now takes tremendous upward swing—often to twice its usual after-meal level. Pancreas overstimulated.
2. Insulin pours out from pancreas. Burns sugar needed, then the rest is stored in the liver as glycogen. Glycogen supply usually ample, sugar converted to fat. You put on weight.
3. Overabundance of insulin still circulates. After three to four hours, hunger pangs start again. Late snack in form of four times as many calories as needed is ingested.
4. Rise to higher peaks of insulin and later on, fall to low levels of sugar again. Process repeats itself in vicious cycle.

You may begin to see what a web of trouble stuffing yourself can cause. Fortunately, your body can offset such effects if they aren't repeated over and over again. This is true of many body functions—if it weren't, I shudder to think of the results! It's the repetition of the stuffing process that's the trap—and it's so easy to let it become a habit. Not only is this habit self-perpetuating, *it trips other mechanisms in your body that tend to make an already bad situation much worse.*

Consider what happens to your elimination processes when you're on the stuffed-up jag. Stuffing over a period of time loads your intestines with vast quantities of waste material. The very aftermath of heavy intakes of food makes you lethargic, as we have already seen. This means the tone of the intestinal muscles is poor; elimination is therefore poor. The products of your body's metabolism pile up, and you are right back where you were a short time ago with the slowing down of metabolism in cells because of the accumulation of wastes, sluggish muscles and brain, and the vicious circle!

Add to this factor of altered metabolism the other common stimulus of overeating and stuffing, nervous tension, and you have double trouble. Without realizing it, you build up tension every day for many reasons. At a certain level (which varies widely with each individual), this nervous build-up must be discharged, *or it may explode into mental disease.*

For some unknown reason, the intestinal tract is the body's favorite target for nervous energy release. When the stomach is stimulated by the large nerves that supply it, hunger pangs result. Hunger pangs cause us to eat, sometimes consciously, sometimes unconsciously. This is often the reason a person who is five feet three inches tall and weighs 200 pounds will be heard to declare that he or she "practically starves" or "never eats much of anything." The person doesn't *realize* it when the box of candy is quickly consumed or that left-over potato salad in the refrigerator disappears—such people are the victims of a cruel game played by their minds in response to nervous tension. Of course, it's better that they overeat than lose their minds. But there is another alternative: *Correct low blood sugar levels* and neither overeat nor lose your mind!

HOW EMOTIONS FREQUENTLY RUN OUT OF CONTROL WITH LOW BLOOD SUGAR CONDITION

Have you ever noticed how some days you seem to flare-up for no apparent reason? Nothing anyone does pleases you; everything goes wrong. Finally, you explode—then, you're "down in the dumps" for the rest of the day or the rest of the week. Frustration causes anger and anger, when it's turned inside, causes depression.

What Causes Frustration

Frustration occurs when anything you're doing doesn't quite work out like you'd like it to. It looms large when at every turn, you've planned wrong, spoken wrong, or acted wrong. On the other hand, it's part of living that we are occassionally thwarted. But morbid frustration—the kind that acts as a real blow to your self-esteem and makes you feel like the proverbial "bottom of a bird cage" needn't be a constant part of your life. Not when you can prevent it from getting this bad *by correcting your low blood sugar!*

When anger and frustration get bad enough to cause depression, your whole system gets out of whack. You can't think, you can't eat, you can't even be sociable. Sometimes, you may even feel as though you might wish to end it all. This is a terrible frame of mind. It's self-destructive and serves neither you nor anyone else any useful purpose.

Case History of Aggravated Frustration

The downcast look on the face of a man I saw recently was all that was really needed to tell the source of his trouble. He came in with his wife who had obviously twisted his arm to get him to seek help. I learned most of the story from his wife since he wasn't up to talking about his troubles.

The husband was always a well-adjusted, reasonably happy and attentive person. He was kind to his family and faithful in his job. About two weeks before this visit, he'd been passed over for a promotion at work. His ordinarily conscientious, hard-driving personality was mortally wounded. About the time of this setback, his wife told me he'd been slowly gaining weight, drinking heavily when arriving home, and never took time for much physical activity. The final blow of not getting his just reward at work was too much. He began to be non-communicative with his family, to neglect his diet, and to start drinking even more than usual. Insomnia soon entered the picture along with the morbid change in his personality. He became a tyrant and frightened his kids as well as his wife.

I soon found out it was useless to try to talk to this man. He didn't want me "poking my nose in his private business" and was more angry than ever with his wife for having brought him to me in the first place. At length, I succeeded in convincing him there was something wrong that we couldn't locate. He agreed to enter the hospital for a short round of tests and, though I didn't mention it then, perhaps a talk with a psychiatrist.

Primarily as a screening move, a blood sugar test was given the man along with some others to rule out disease. To my surprise, the sugar curve was hypoglycemic—he had a pronounced *low blood sugar curve*. His sugar curve was the only abnormal part of his examination. Furthermore, he wanted no part of any "head-shrinkers," and I couldn't persuade him to talk even once with a psychiatrist.

Results of Special Diet

In desperation, I tried the only approach I had left. I placed him on six feedings a day and a special diet designed to furnish normal amounts of proteins, carbohydrates and fat, yet also designed to cause weight loss. I didn't allow him any visitors except his wife, from whom I extracted a promise not to bring food or drink of any kind during her visits. At bedtime and in the morning I had glucagon, the drug that increases sugar levels, given him routinely. I also talked the physiotherapy department, fortunately headed by a male technician who was a staunch supporter of physical conditioning, into working this man out three times a day for about one half hour. By the end of three days, he was sleeping like a log without sedation. At the end of five days, he had lost eight pounds of weight and would chat with me on rounds easily and without strain.

He went home in a week 12 pounds lighter, on his way to the best physical condition his muscles had been in since high school and eager to get back to his job and family. His blood sugar curve returned to normal!

Later this man confided in me that the job promotion was well deserved for the other man who got it, but he just couldn't seem to forget the fact that he'd somehow failed. He also said that as he looked back on his time of trouble, he had to laugh at his foolish behavior.

HOW TO BRIGHTEN UP THOSE "BLACK-OUTS"

The "black-out" of a person has been a medical enigma for centuries. There are a good many causes for black-out spells; some of them can be traced to low blood sugar, others to high blood sugar, and still others seem to have nothing at all to do with blood sugar. A black-out is anything that causes a loss of consciousness.

Therefore, if you get clobbered on the head hard enough, you have a black-out. If you faint, you have a black-out. If you have epilepsy, you are subject to black-outs. When you're asleep, you're blacked-out in a very real sense. With the possible exception of sleep, the three immediate causes of black-outs are a sudden decrease in the amount of blood flowing to the brain, hypoglycemia (low blood sugar), and a blow to the head.

With ordinary fainting, a decrease in the blood flow to your brain is the cause. Some people faint more easily than others, but the problem is the same—the great vessels in your neck control the blood flow to your brain. If anything happens to upset this control, which is done through a special set of nerves, the pressure and therefore the amount of blood to your brain is suddenly cut down for a very short period of time. You faint, pass out, or have a black-out, whatever you wish to call it.

The process of getting up from a bed or chair to a standing position calls for changes in this blood regulation. The older you are, the slower this change can be made. This is why older people sometimes feel woozy or dizzy when they stand up too quickly. The point is that what I said earlier applies: Your brain *must have a constant supply of oxygen and sugar to perform its work.*

When you receive a rap on the head, you may be knocked out. In the prize-fighting business, many people are knocked out by a blow to the jaw. Since the jaw is directly connected to the head, a black-out can occur with a sufficiently hard blow to it. The cause of this type of black-out is the concussion that the brain cells get when the head is struck. There is a sudden diminishing of blood in and around the brain cells, and unconsciousness is the result.

The hypoglycemic or low blood sugar black-out occurs when the blood sugar falls rapidly to quite low levels. Some people can stand more of this sugar fall than others. Low blood sugar black-outs can result in convulsions (fits) just like epilepsy, and to see one person with a convulsion from epilepsy and another having a fit from low blood sugar is to see exactly the same thing.

Signs of Falling Blood Sugar

When your blood sugar falls rapidly, you notice a cold clammy feeling all over your body. The pupils of your eyes grow larger, making them sensitive to light that ordinarily wouldn't bother them. Your pulse rate goes up—you may have palpitations like our little lady in the emergency room I mentioned previously. You then notice a symptom very specific for low blood sugar black-outs: You get very shaky and jittery—at this point, you may black-out. When you wake up seconds or a minute or two later, you may have some difficulty remembering what happened, where you are, or even what day it is. Such is the way of low blood sugar black-outs.

The hypoglycemic black-out is dangerous, especially if there are convulsions (fits) with it. For this reason, it is well to seek medical help if convulsions have occurred with such black-outs. If they haven't, but black-outs have occurred, you can easily terminate a black-out before it happens simply by eating or drinking anything rich in carbohydrate like sugared fruit juice or bread with lots of butter and jelly on it. Just plain table sugar will suffice in lieu of anything else. Remember that the sugar or carbohydrate must be taken *at the first sign of the low blood sugar attack*.

It's also a must for all diabetics (the condition of too much blood sugar), whether they take injections of insulin or one of the pill forms of anti-diabetic medicines, that low blood sugar be carefully prevented. This is especially true in children whose requirements for insulin and sugar vary widely from day to day. It can become a tragedy if an unconscious or semi-conscious person —a known diabetic—is delivered to a hospital if it is assumed that the person is in diabetic coma—he may well be in insulin or hypoglycemic shock. To treat him with massive doses of insulin could be irreversibly harmful. I've seen this happen enough times in busy hospitals to know that it is a real problem. The last case I saw was a patient of a colleague friend of mine who wasn't called when the diabetic child was delivered in a comatose (unconscious) state to the emergency room of a hospital. The house doctor assumed diabetic coma and treated with large doses of insulin, including a whopping dose intravenously. It turned out to be the opposite case—the child had taken too much insulin and hadn't covered it adequately with carbohydrate. He was in low sugar shock, and suffered brain damage as a result of prolonged low blood sugar.

In the last year, I've encountered three men who were picked up on the streets, staggering and incoherent, who were assumed to be drunk by the police. They were consequently put in the local jail. In all three cases, there was permanent brain damage from delay in treating the extremely low blood sugar conditions. They will never be the same again, and will probably become permanent wards of the state.

Every day, alcoholics withdrawing from liquor are picked up in large cities for creating disturbances. A large number of these people are headed either for delirium tremens, commonly known as "the DT's," or for convulsions as a result of alcoholic withdrawal. They "dry out" in very poor surroundings, often in "drunk tanks" located in the dirtiest, most poorly staffed portions of local jails. What these people need, all other considerations aside as to their undesirability or why they have become alcoholics, is sugar administered intravenously. If they don't get it, they can, and often do, sustain the same kind of brain damage described above. I'll have more to say about the problem of the alcoholic later in this book.

HOW MOST ACHING BACKS AND PAINFUL JOINTS CAN BE ALLEVIATED

Next to the common headache, the painful muscle and joint with aches and spasms must be the most common symptom complex in the world. Like the headache, no one seems perfectly immune to this distressing, sometimes crippling, malady.

You can prevent 90 per cent of the agony from these symptoms by attention to low blood sugar.

How to Relieve Your Painful Back

Low back muscle and ligament strain is the most common cause for lumbago and arthralgia of the back. Because your back muscles and ligaments are so large compared to others in the body, when they're strained or overstretched, they hurt more and for longer periods of time than strains in any other area of your anatomy.

There is no more neglected spot than your back. Physical conditioning programs generally forget the back exists, and it suffers because of it. This neglect, combined with the fact that people fail to use common sense when lifting, straining or carrying heavy objects, accounts for the vast majority of backaches. Add to the fact that in the human animal, the back is basically unstable because of his relatively recent switch to walking upright, and you have a problem in mechanics.

Strains of back muscles and ligaments are predisposed by poor conditioning. Poor conditioning makes muscles and ligaments soft, have poor cell metabolism, and accumulate waste products. Does this sound familiar? We've already seen how these factors result from low blood sugar. The back is no exception.

I've taught many people how to deal with their aching backs using nothing more than conditioning and proper nourishment. To this routine, I usually add instructions on how to properly lift, carry, and push and pull heavy objects. Very few people fail to improve under this therapy. A good many people would if they take the time to learn.

The Painful Joint

Painful joints are a scourge to mankind. A list of causes for arthritis, the term that means inflammation in or around a joint, is almost endless. So are cures and modes of therapy—every five to ten years, a treatment plan is hauled out of the dusty closet of "tried and true" methods used a generation ago. Usually, with the same disappointing results.

The current thought of the medical profession is that arthritis is a combination of two main factors—heredity and stress. This disease is like many others in that you may be born with certain factors in the make-up of your cells that predispose to arthritis, but it takes a precipitating or stressful factor to actually bring on the trouble. It's like a train. A train consists of an engine and a number of joined boxcars. If you merely join together the boxcars, there isn't a train until it's joined to the engine. Similarly, if you have just the engine, there isn't a complete train until it's hooked up to the coaches.

It seems reasonable, therefore, to work on that part of the combination that has to do with stress, since none of us can do much about his heredity. The way to develop resistance to stress is to get yourself into the most efficient state of mechanical well-being possible. The way to this goal is through physical conditioning and diet, as well as keeping yourself as free as possible from disease states and mental imbalance. It will come as no surprise, in view of what we've already talked about, that your body's response to stress is hinged on two factors: your endocrine glands and your nervous system. It can be taken almost as a certainty that whenever your endocrine system is involved in a response from whatever stimulus, blood sugar levels are involved.

Of the hundreds of patients I've seen with arthritis, virtually all of them had undue physical and mental trauma in their backgrounds. And though it's true that one can't avoid physical and mental trauma in his life, he can start on a preventive program such that when the trauma comes, his body is better able to cope efficiently with it.

The Painful Ligament and Tendon

Ligaments are the short gristle pieces of tissue that hold bones together at any joint. Wherever there is a joint, there are ligaments that hold it together. They're involved in strains, sprains, and arthritis, along with the cartilage that cushions the bones making up the joints. They, too, respond to conditioning.

Tendons are the long pieces of tissue that anchor a muscle to a bone at its beginning and end. As you look at the back of your hand and wiggle your fingers, the rippling beneath the skin is caused by some of the hand muscle tendons. They are subject to strain and inflammation and also respond to conditioning.

A Case of Surgery Not the Whole Answer

A patient who had back surgery for a disc rupture once said to me that he expected to be crippled for the rest of his life. His injury was accidental, and the small piece of cartilage that cushions the bones of the back had been damaged and was pressing on an important nerve going down into his leg. Surgery removed the offending piece of cartilage and fused that part of his back left unstable by the disc removal. But it hadn't cured his back pain.

The man was unable to resume his former job as a construction worker because of continuing pain and distress in his low back. In examining this man's back, it was obvious what had happened. For some time before surgery, and for a long time afterward, he had to be restricted from doing anything that might strain his back. This is a necessary evil in dealing with injury to any joint— it takes a long time for nature to heal the area following surgery. But at the same time, the ligaments, tendons and muscles also suffer from lack of use. They become soft, easily strained, and *predisposed to poor sugar utilization*. When the healing process is finished, they need re-conditioning. And that's just what this man hadn't done.

When, under harsh protest, I put this man on a graduated series of back exercises and blood sugar control through dietary habits, and with control of the pain I knew would follow for awhile, by using mild analgesics (pain-relieving drugs), he gradually improved. It took about four months to get this man over the hump—remember the back is slow to come around at best and the muscles and ligaments are large. But he was able to resume his former job. He hasn't had any more injuries, fortunately, and can now do anything he used to do without discomfort.

It's a shame that this difficult but almost always present critical period is neglected following surgery or other trauma. The patient with a bad back is usually in limbo and is generally disliked by everybody because of his chronically distressing dilemma.

HOW TO RECHARGE YOUR YOUTH WITH LOW BLOOD SUGAR REVERSAL

In every animal species there is a biological average maximum for his lifespan. Man is no exception. Man's "three-score and ten" is his average maximum, and hard facts indicate that no matter where he lives or under what conditions, he will succumb between 70–75 years.

At this point, I'm not especially concerned with the question whether man can be made or should be made to live longer. I'm concerned with the people I'm sure you know who look ten or fifteen years older than their actual age—the problem of *premature* aging. Nutritionists have come a long way in recent years in identifying the factors that cause cells in the human body to age. As it stands now, there are several things that seem to cause aging in the human cell. One of these stands out as vitally important. This factor is the one having to do with the efficiency with which waste products within the individual cell are disposed of. It has been clearly shown that the human cell becomes filled with "clinkers"—masses of waste material that can't be eliminated —and that these clinkers clog the cell, robbing it of its capacity to perform even its basic metabolic functions, not to speak of its particular specific function, such as the brain cell that is involved with your thinking process or a heart muscle cell that is involved with keeping your heart beating.

Scientists are today about ready to be able to tell from a small specimen of your skin, for instance, how many of these cells are so clogged with "clinkers" that they are for practical purposes dead or useless. From this information, they can predict with accuracy how many of the other cells in your body are similarly affected. In short, it will soon be possible to see how much a person has actually aged, based on information obtained from a few of that person's skin cells.

Wouldn't it be nice if one could at least prevent this *premature* aging? You can! By paying close attention to your blood sugar control.

Case History of a Man Who Looked Much Older Than His Real Age

It's one thing to appear, but not *feel,* older than you really are, but it's an unfortunate situation when you both feel and look older than your chronological age. Such was the plight of a 45-year-old man I know. He looked about 60, while his wife looked her true age of 42.

He had been a chronic alcoholic for a number of years in his late 20's and 30's, but had long since been on the wagon. He'd sustained a small amount of liver damage, but not enough to cause his present plight, which was simply that he felt he was losing everything he had, including the love of his wife and family, and that he would probably pass out of the picture before he reached 50.

This man "de-aged" in response to the following changes in his blood sugar control:

1. *A complete revision of his diet with added vitamins.* He had sustained nutritional starvation so long during his

period of alcoholism that his body was beginning to deteriorate.

2. *A 20 minute, three times a day routine of graduated exercise.* His protein depletion had become so severe that his muscles were wasting away.

3. *A change in his life's activity such that fresh air and vigorous exertion became a daily habit.* Vacations were always taken in the mountains or woods, rather than the plush places where he just sat around and was waited on all day.

4. *The start of an avocation in addition to his business, which happened to be sales.* He had once been quite a tinkerer. He started to build scale models of the world's great bridges and soon became an authority in this field. He has since exhibited his models at engineering conventions.

Instead of a pale, dry, wrinkled skin, this man now has a healthful pink glow to his smooth skinned cheeks. He is slim and trim instead of fat and flabby as he had become. He is vigorous and has energy to spare rather than lazy. His personality has changed from that of early senility to a youthful, energetic extroverted type with many worthwhile goals. He is a very useful contributing member of society, whereas before he was, in his own words, completely worthless.

SUMMARY

1. Many of life's "small aggravations" are tied to low blood sugar. A combination of two or more of these aggravations figure in the majority of all ill-health, non-productivity, unhappiness, and eventual disease. Start to control them now before they get a chance to start.

2. Mind and body functions are always and at all times interconnected. What happens to your body can't avoid affecting your mind, and mental trouble always affects your body. Blood sugar control affects both mind and body to the good, regardless of which pole, mind or body, you work with.

3. If there is doubt whether one or a set of symptoms you may have is a reflection of disease, seek medical help. If things come out normal after a medical check-up, expect low blood sugar

control to improve your health and start you on your way to really living again.

4. The majority of the "blues" headaches, black-outs, and back-aches are traced to poor blood sugar control. Sometimes, such symptoms spell trouble. Learn to tell those that require help from those you can correct—and start today correcting them!

5. If you're getting "too soon old and too late smart," as the old Dutch saying goes, correcting low blood sugar will head off a pack of troubles for you later.

3

How to Reverse Negative Metabolism
for More Vigorous Health

We've talked a good deal about your physical condition thus far. Now I'm going to start you on your way to doing something about it. The first place to start is with your weight—the keystone of blood sugar control and vigorous health.

If you have a state of *negative metabolism,* you have no control over low blood sugar. *If you don't have control over low blood sugar, you don't have, and can never have, good health.* Negative metabolism, as we shall see, is any condition in which your energy turnover is not working well. Negative metabolism encompasses both over and underweight states and may even be present in the face of normal weight.

Both your endocrine glands, the ones that control your body's vital functions, and your state of mind are affected by the metabolism of the cells they're made up of—if metabolism is out of control, so will your endocrine glands and brain refuse to function properly.

Since your metabolism is dependent upon what you eat as well as how you eat, we will look at these items and their control in this chapter.

HOW TO SIZE UP YOUR METABOLIC CONDITION

I'm sure you've often wondered what kind of physical condition you might be in. Perhaps you sense that it isn't good right now, and you're probably right! I find that most people have neglected their bodies as well as their minds. *This is why so many people have low blood sugar symptoms.*

Extend your arms. Look at the under surfaces of them. Do the muscles hang limply and quiver on movement like jello? Stand up and look down at your feet. Can you see them clearly without sucking in your belly? For that matter, can you suck in your abdomen? If you can't, you're in negative metabolism.

At your office or when you're in town and must go in an office building, do you ride the elevator or take the stairs? When you have an errand to run, do you walk or ride a bike or do you take the family car? If you consistently ride the elevator or ride in your car on errands within reasonable walking distance, try it the other way next time. If you find yourself huffing and puffing at the top of the stairs or on arrival at the store, you're *not* in reasonable physical condition.

Consult the weight table and see how you fit with the index of healthful weight.

How do you stack up? If you're like most people, you've probably got some work to do! If you're wondering about how to judge whether you have a small, medium, or large frame, judge it from the size of the bones that make up your skeleton and the size of your muscles (not your flab!). For men, if size small shirts fit you well, your frame is usually small; if size medium shirts fit, your frame is medium, and if you must wear large shirts to fit properly, your frame is usually large. For women, your shell or T-neck sizes may be used to gauge your frames in the same way.

In using the height-weight-frame tables, you should *not* exceed the maximum figure in your particular category. It is permissible to carry 10 per cent *less* weight for your height and frame than the *minimum* range given for each category, however. It has re-

MEN
25 and older

HEIGHT WITH SHOES Feet Inches	SMALL FRAME Pounds	MEDIUM FRAME	LARGE FRAME
5 2	112–120	118–129	126–141
5 3	115–123	121–133	129–144
5 4	118–126	124–136	132–148
5 5	121–129	127–139	135–152
5 6	124–133	130–143	138–156
5 7	128–137	134–147	142–161
5 8	132–141	138–152	147–166
5 9	136–145	142–156	151–170
5 10	140–150	146–160	155–174
5 11	144–154	150–165	159–179
6 0	148–158	154–170	164–184
6 1	152–162	158–175	168–189
6 2	156–167	162–180	173–194
6 3	160–171	167–185	178–199
6 4	164–175	172–190	182–204

WOMEN
25 and older

HEIGHT WITH SHOES 2 inch heels Feet Inches	SMALL FRAME Pounds	MEDIUM FRAME	LARGE FRAME
4 10	92– 98	96–107	104–107
4 11	94–101	98–110	106–122
5 0	96–104	101–113	109–125
5 1	99–107	104–116	112–128
5 2	102–110	107–119	115–131
5 3	105–113	110–122	118–134
5 4	108–116	113–126	121–138
5 5	111–119	116–130	125–142
5 6	114–123	120–135	129–146
5 7	118–127	124–139	133–150
5 8	122–131	128–143	137–154
5 9	126–135	132–147	141–158
5 10	130–140	136–151	145–163
5 11	134–144	140–155	149–168
6 0	138–148	144–159	153–173

cently been shown, in fact, by careful studies conducted by the nation's life insurance companies, that carrying about 10 per cent less weight than the standards given in the tables gives you increased chances for a longer, healthier life.

MIRRORS DON'T LIE ABOUT YOUR HEALTH

A careful objective look at yourself in your mirror will tell you the final story. As you stand facing your mirror, look carefully at your face. Are your jowls (skin around your jaws and lower cheeks) hanging down in folds? How about beneath your eyes— are there rolling folds of skin hanging down beneath dark circles? If so, assume you need attention to blood sugar levels. Next, look at your chest. The pectoral muscles are those large muscles on either side of your breast bone behind the nipples. Men's pectorals should be firm enough when relaxed to take up all sag at the breast and nipple areas. Women's breasts, which are suspended from their pectorals, should not sag down onto the chest wall or abdomen. Tissues should be firm and the breast should stand out from the chest wall equally as much at the bottoms as at the tops.

Now focus on your abdomen. Is it flat from the end of your breast bone to your pubic bone below your navel? It should be. How about the taper of your abdomen? Your waist line should be narrower than either chest or hips. Next, turn to the side and look at your profile. Head tilted forward and shoulders slumped? Upper part of your back curve outwardly? Lower back curved inward? They shouldn't be. Does loose fat hang from the buttock areas? If so, you've got some correction of that low blood sugar to start!

For every one of you who do the mirror test and consult the weight tables and find yourself underweight and presenting a scrawny appearance, at least 1,000 or more of you will find the opposite to be true. In either case, you can correct the problem without drugs or special apparatus and without the advantage of a therapist and a gymnasium at hand to guide you. Just remember that it's the low blood sugar villain you're after. The weight and the image you see in the mirror will correct themselves if you set as your goal the *total correction of blood sugar levels.*

THE DO'S AND DON'TS OF DIETING

The following rules should be committed to memory to help guide you in dieting:

1. *Never eat until you're full.* This applies to overweight and underweights alike. If you're losing weight, one of the things that must be done is that your stomach must shrink. You can't shrink it by distending it to its fullest measure at each meal. As your stomach shrinks, your appetite will automatically decrease.

2. *Don't go to the table at any meal feeling either upset or ravenously hungry.* Form the habit of eating six smaller meals a day if you can. This can be done by cutting down on the sizes and kinds of food at breakfast, lunch and dinner and adding a snack at mid-morning, mid-afternoon and at bedtime. This way, main meals are approached with a reasonable appetite, but not with your blood sugar levels so low that you have to eat three times as much as you should.

   Being emotionally upset at mealtime spells trouble. Digestion is poorly performed, food is taken without much regard for what's in it, and you generally end up by overeating.

3. *Cut out of your diet completely 75 per cent of the carbohydrates you are used to eating.* Carbohydrates, remember, are broken down to sugar and stored as fat if not needed. It's from carbohydrates, not fat, that the bulk of your excess weight comes. This isn't to say that you should feel free to eat all the fat you want—just trim away half the fat on meat and eat the rest. But do switch to skim milk in drinking and for cooking and do switch to polyunsaturated spreads (margarine) in cooking and baking for use on bread and toast. Carbohydrates are high in all frying, cooking and salad oils. Stop using them! Bread, potatoes, pastries, spaghetti and macaroni—all the starchy foods, in other words—are quite high in carbohydrates. Divide the usual portion of such foods on your plate in four equal

parts—put back *three* of these four portions and eat the remaining portion. You can make up part of your remaining appetite by eating protein. (Protein also contains calories, but only half the amount by weight as carbohydrates.) Proteins are found in high amounts in all meat, fish, fowl and cheeses. Leguminous vegetables—those that grow in pods like corn and beans—also are high in protein. Form the habit of skipping desserts entirely.

4. *Cut your liquor intake in half.* Alcohol is a dietary carbohydrate as far as your metabolism is concerned. A martini may contain as many as 250 to 300 calories—as many calories as you need for one entire meal! Don't misunderstand, I'm not a teetotaler in any sense of the word. Proper intake of alcoholic beverages exerts a very beneficial effect which I'll explain later. At this point in your blood sugar control, however, you must get your weight in line, and overconsumption of alcohol is one habit that will absolutely stop your effort in effective control of blood sugar levels.

5. *Use only sugar substitutes in coffee and cereals or in cooking and baking.* Table sugar is, as we have seen, pure unadulterated carbohydrate in its simplest form. What we are trying to do here is to force your body to burn up its stored fat and carbohydrate and, in turn, reduce your weight. If you keep giving your body all it needs of immediate energy in the form of sugar, it doesn't bother to burn up your fat, and you fail to lose weight.

On hot days or for snacks, avoid using soda pop, candy and sweetened iced drinks unless they are the low-calorie kind. Use one of the artificial sweeteners. They contain no calories and can't upset your main goal: *the control of low blood sugar.*

HOW TO CONTROL THOSE "CONTRARY" CALORIES

I've referred a couple of times to the word "calorie," but haven't dwelt on the word in describing how to diet. I don't intend to. The reason for this is that I think calories and calorie counting are greatly overdone. If you have to make a complicated calculation before each meal or before taking a snack, it has been my experience that interest in dieting is soon lost.

Calories are the specific units of energy contained in a given amount of food. I can still remember the days when one had to sit down with a calorie chart and a food scale and carefully figure out the exact amount and kinds of foods he had to eat that meal if he were trying to lose weight or if he had diabetes and took insulin. This practice has become a thing of the past. You don't have to know anything at all about calories, let alone count them each time you eat, to lose weight.

The only thing you have to remember about calories is that you must ingest fewer of them than you burn up each day if you're to lose weight and control your sugar levels. The five rules just given will insure this. In an appendix at the end of this book, you will find sample diets for reducing.

You need not fear that you will short your body on carbohydrates while dieting. Your body metabolism will automatically take out of storage the carbohydrate your diet doesn't supply. If you make your body do this over a period of time, you can't help losing weight. On the other hand, if you constantly supply carbohydrates your body doesn't use over a period of time, you can't help *gaining* weight.

It may seem something of a contradiction that restricting sugar as you must do while dieting would help in controlling the levels of low blood sugar. But remember that previously you had to take in too much sugar in order to become overweight, and it is this overweight that is causing you your troubles with low blood sugar now!

Of all the factors that have to do with your blood sugar control, *too much weight is the most likely reason you aren't able to control your blood sugar levels.*

HOW CRIPPLING DISEASE CAN BE AVOIDED BY SLIMMING DOWN

You really owe it to your heart, your lungs, your blood vessels, your brain and your joints to make it possible for them to function well for you until the end of your life span. It's impossible to describe the agony and the pain that people must endure in their mid and later lives when they let their blood sugar control get so far out of hand that their obesity brings on the ravages of disease. I can say without reservation that fully 90 per cent of all the disease that afflicts mankind today can be greatly modified or prevented with proper attention to blood sugar control earlier in life.

Take your joints, for example. They definitely weren't designed to carry and support weight outside the upper ranges given for you in the height-weight tables previously set out. If you force joints to continually support excess weight, the only thing to expect is that those joints will degenerate. And when they do, they can't be replaced.

The relationship between being overweight and heart and blood vessel disease can't be overemphasized. If anything, the problem is underestimated. People with too much weight have more circulating fats in their bloodstream than is normal. This fat deposits on the inside linings of blood vessels and starts "plaques" on their walls. These "plaques" are calcified by the system and soon plug up the vessels so blood can't pass through the vessel as it should. When a coronary heart attack occurs, it is just such a plugged-up vessel in the heart muscle that causes it. When a stroke occurs, it is the rupture or plugging of just such a blood vessel in the brain that causes it. When the circulation in one of your legs starts to shut off causing severe pain when you walk a few hundred feet, it's just such a plugged vessel that causes it.

You can prevent all this, and a lot more besides, by controlling your blood sugar levels *now*. The way to start is by peeling off those pounds *now*.

The fact that you may already have suffered some of the disease states brought on by low blood sugar need not discourage you or cause you to feel glum. This vicious process can be halted even if you've let it go longer than you should have.

The point is that if you're already too heavy and have had symptoms of disease, you are in the middle of a circle that will grow larger the longer you put off doing something about it. Obesity causes even lower levels of blood sugar. This causes a string of reactions that make you eat even more. This, in turn, makes the depths of blood sugar greater. Disease not only increases, but life shortens with each passing year of poor blood sugar control. You may well add years of healthful life to your span in spite of the fact that you've neglected your diet altogether. Start today with a goal of longer happier living with blood sugar control!

WHAT TO DO IF UNDERWEIGHT

If you find your weight is down in excess of 10 per cent of the minimum range for your height and frame in the tables, your problem is just the opposite of the overweight person, and fortunately, far less serious. People who are simply thin and high-strung are often labeled as having weak constitutions. This is not necessarily so. If you've been so labeled, your constitution may be as strong as the next—perhaps stronger! Your trouble is very much like the patient I spoke of previously whom I saw in the emergency room who was frail and weak all her life because that's the way she was raised. She overcame her weak constitution, and so can you.

Daily Diet Guidelines

The following guidelines should be a part of your everyday routine in diet matters.

1. *Eat until you are comfortably full.* Don't become stuffed, as described earlier in this chapter, but do eat approximately 20 per cent more food than usual each day. Your problem, unlike the overweight person, is that you need to *gently* stretch your stomach which has become too small for your good health.
2. *Snack at least three times a day.* Your snacks are taken for similar reasons as for those who are reducing, but you needn't be concerned about carbohydrate at this point. Roll them in by eating more of the foods recommended to be cut back for the overweight problem. Use plenty of real sugar in coffee, tea and cereals, but be careful not to snack on pure carbohydrate foods *by themselves.* Use carbohydrate, protein and fats together, even with snacks, so that you don't drive down your blood sugar levels as in the earlier example in this chapter for the obese person.

3. *Be certain that you are absorbing what you eat.* It isn't uncommon that underweight problems are coupled with poor digestion and poor absorption after digestion. If you don't seem to be making headway with your problem after a reasonable time, consult a medical expert. He'll make certain tests to see if your body is handling foodstuffs properly. It's a good idea to take extra vitamins and minerals while trying to lose, as well as trying to gain, weight. This can be done quite cheaply and efficiently by using Brewer's yeast tablets, eating plenty of fruit rind (there is often more vitamin C in fruit rind than in the fruit itself), and by drinking plenty of milk—skimmed, if you are losing weight, extra high fat milk if you want to gain.

Above all, don't be discouraged in spite of past failures you may have experienced. Your organism may be specially constructed to be of small stature and frame. You only need to strive, remember, for a goal of within 10 per cent of the minimum weight for your frame and height. Once there, you've overcome a mighty obstacle in your blood sugar control.

POSITIVE METABOLISM AND ENDOCRINE BALANCE

Every one of your vital endocrine glands is affected by negative metabolism. This is especially true of obesity. Following is a brief description of these glands and their functions.

1. *Pituitary gland.* You now have learned that the pituitary gland is the master gland of all the other glands in the body. In conditions of overweight, the pituitary gland is depressed. One of the many functions of this amazing gland is that it figures in the use of sugar by the cell—it inhibits indiscriminate burning up of energy by the cell until insulin comes along to release the cell's machinery that burns sugar. If the pituitary is deactivated, so to speak, by an overweight condition, insulin will tend to overact and there results . . . yes, low blood sugar! Since the pituitary also exerts control over the glands of reproduction, it's not surprising to find fat people suffering from lack of

sexual capacity and, in women, from disturbances in their menstrual cycle.

2. *Thyroid gland.* This gland is the cell energy gland. It controls the *rate* of utilization of sugar by the cells, presuming the sugar and the insulin levels are in normal balance. In the state of obesity, this gland sometimes slows down, often to a standstill. This can only mean one thing: Increased deposition by your body of sugar and carbohydrate (since the cell can't use it) as fat. And the cycle worsens! More fat—more excess carbohydrate deposited—slower metabolism, etc.

3. *Pancreas gland.* You now know that this gland produces insulin—that necessary chemical needed by the cell to burn energy. In the case of the fat person, this gland tends to be overstimulated in an effort by your body to rid itself of all the carbohydrate. But its efforts are thwarted! Your pituitary and thyroid are working against it. It fails to do the job. Result? Again, our nemesis, low blood sugar levels!

4. *Adrenal glands.* The adrenals are the alert glands, as you've already learned. Among other things, your adrenals stimulate the liver to release glycogen (carbohydrate) that can raise low blood sugar states. But, again, in the fat body, the adrenals are depressed by the lowered efficiency of the pituitary under whose control the adrenals remain. Result? No glycogen, and no correction of the low blood sugar state.

These results of obesity on your endocrine glands just have to do with their roles in metabolism. Is it any wonder, with all these glands out of adjustment, that so many disease states result? Think of it! Through the mere act of reducing, you're remedying the entire machinery of your body's inner workings!

WHAT TO DO ABOUT THAT NAGGING APPETITE

The first thing on the minds of most people when they decide to lose or gain weight is what can be taken to eliminate their nagging appetites. I fear this is altogether too often the way we've become conditioned to deal with problems: To just take a pill and somehow, magically, or through the miracle of modern science, the problem for which the drug is taken is spirited away.

What we've all forgotten, apparently, and this includes we physicians as well, is that drugs are not without their toxic effects and side reactions, and their use always needs to be tempered with a sober look at the question: What will this drug do to the patient's system that may be harmful? Appetite drugs are no exception. In my opinion, none of the many drugs used to control appetite have any place whatsoever in diet control management. This may sound peculiar, but my experience has been, and what I've seen of others' experience bears it out completely, that such drugs do much more harm than good, and for this reason their use in appetite suppression should be abandoned altogether!

There are many reasons for my attitude about these drugs. First and foremost, all appetite drugs are habit-forming. Since dieting takes a long time in many cases, no drug that is habit-forming should ever be used. Secondly, all such drugs are stimulants to the nervous system. They cause overstimulation with nervousness, irritability and insomnia, and they stimulate the pancreas gland to oversecrete insulin with the results we've just finished talking about—low blood sugar levels. You're trying to reverse this process! As if these reasons were not sufficient, it's well known that many of today's youth use these drugs to produce euphoria. One of the most often named drugs in use by young people today as I see them coming into the mental health hospital where I work is "speed" or "crystal," slang names for the drug Benzedrine, a commonly used family of medicines for appetite control. Some of these youngsters even dissolve the "reducing pills" in water and inject the drug into their veins!

Appetite Control Drugs and Low Blood Sugar Levels

The most important thing to remember about appetite control drugs is that they drive down your blood sugar levels. The very thing we're striving to correct! Even if they did help control your appetite for a time, using them invariably ends with more problems than you started with. The most important place for all such drugs is in their containers.

Drugless Appetite Controls

What you *can* do about helping control your appetite is set forth as follows:

1. There are a number of simple, *bulk-forming* compounds available. These substances are *not* drugs, nor do they have any other action than forming a harmless glob in your stomach when combined with water. This glob will often control those hunger pangs when they become tough. These inert materials do not require a prescription. Just follow the directions on the label. They exert no other action or effect whatsoever. Ask your doctor about them.

2. Starting the routine of eating five or six meals a day by itself often allows you to be rid of annoying hunger pangs. Hunger generally occurs between meals. If you've followed the diet rules given earlier in this section, your routine calls for proper snacks.

3. There are a number of foods that don't add much of anything to nutrition in general and certainly not carbohydrate. These foods can aid you in control of your appetite. Such foods are lettuce, celery, greens (spinach, turnip, collard) from the leafy vegetables, potato peelings, fruit rinds, rye crisp, and melba toast. Taken with liberal amounts of water or skim milk, these can control hunger pangs quite well. I've found that when starting on a diet, you may expect to have some discomfort with hunger pangs (appetite stimulation) for four to six weeks. After this, you may expect them to be gone completely, and your diet will follow without difficulty even though you have by this time reduced your total food intake as much as 60 per cent.

HOW TO KEEP YOUR POSITIVE METABOLISM THROUGHOUT LIFE

I've been asked many times if aging doesn't add problems to dieting, or if one's diet doesn't change a good deal with advancing years. The answer to both these questions is "no." It's true that with years, your metabolism changes somewhat. You don't require the energy, for one thing, to carry on your lives. *But, your blood sugar levels still need to be regulated, perhaps more strongly than ever when you pass the 50 year mark.* For this reason, dieting for overweight is even more important at this later time of life.

The same rules apply with older age and dieting as with younger ages. One thing seems certain with advancing years—the closer you are to your normal weight range in the height-weight-frame tables in this book, the healthier you'll stay!

It's generally a tougher job to change your weight if you're past 55 or 60 years. This is because your metabolism has slowed down compared to what it was at, say, age 25–30 years. This is natural, though, and you needn't be discouraged from doing what your scales tell you needs to be done. You'll be glad you did!

Elimination of Wastes

Remember those cell "clinkers" mentioned earlier? The products of waste that pile up in your cells with age? Well, those wastes need to be inhibited and eliminated. That's why it's important that a well-established routine of diet and exercise be at hand with aging. In addition, with aging comes a stronger need for vitamins and minerals. The sources I listed previously are as good as any. Elimination becomes more of a problem with aging because of a slowing of physical activity and loss of tone of the abdominal muscles, and because of this, a loss of muscle tone in the intestinal tract. More than ever, with aging, you need good control of blood sugar levels through good habits of diet and exercise and good habits of mind. When you pass age 45, pay even more attention to weight. If it isn't where it should be, take the necessary steps. Plan to spend at least an hour a day doing some kind of exercise. Walking, hiking, housework, swimming, or one of the simple routines covered in the next chapter. You'll be a new person for your efforts.

HOW TO FORM GOOD NUTRITION HABITS

The following general rules will help insure your constant nutritional regulation consistent with optimum blood sugar regulation.

PROTEIN. It's quite difficult to overdo protein intake. Protein buildup and breakdown in your body goes on more rapidly than any other process of metabolism. Your diet should, without exception, consist of at least twice the amount of protein as carbohydrate, and four times the amount of protein as fats.

Remember, your body has the means by which to change protein into carbohydrate, should the need arise. This is an automatic process and will go on continually and regularly without special attention on your part. As you bring your blood sugar levels under more and more control, your need for protein increases. Protein is essential for your muscle health, as well as for virtually all the processes that your endocrine glands must perform. The chemicals that these vital glands make for the vast regulation of your body's machinery are *all basically made of protein*. Eat protein with gusto and in high quantities in your diet.

During periods of body stress, protein is even more important, and is usually the hardest item in your diet to replenish because of poor appetite. During the period immediately after surgery, for instance, your body must have huge amounts of protein to mend the operative site and to maintain muscle tone. The same is true during and after a bout with pneumonia, with a heart attack, or with a mental breakdown. If you must, during these periods of stress *force* yourself to eat extra protein between and during mealtimes. Your body needs it!

CARBOHYDRATE. Regulating carbohydrate intake is absolutely essential to losing weight. It's equally essential *to continue regulating carbohydrates* after ideal weight levels are reached. Do not use over half the amounts of carbohydrates in your diet as you use protein. You don't have to weigh and measure foodstuffs to achieve good balance in your diet. Remember to learn to inspect the amount of food that is on your plate. If the amounts aren't balanced as you look at your plate, *remove the excess carbohydrate* from it. Put those extra potatoes, slices of bread, and most of that gravy back in their dishes! Of course carbohydrate is essential, but it's the overuse of it that has gotten your blood sugar out of control. Your body is marvelously adapted to store carbohydrate for future use. When you looked in the mirror earlier, you saw the results of stored carbohydrates hanging down as flab from your muscles and skin. Pare this flab off beginning today.

Exercise in any form, especially if it's more than you're used to, does put a demand on your body for more carbohydrate for immediate use as cell energy. When you begin to increase your physical activities after reading the next chapter, you'll begin to see just how much of this extra energy your body requires to maintain blood sugar levels. Take in just enough carbohydrate to satisfy this demand—and no more. You'll be surprised how easy it is to gauge how much you should take—your body will let you know through your appetite and through some of the signs of low blood sugar you have learned. Learn to read these messages carefully.

FATS. Fats are the enigma of nutrition. Contrary to what we used to think, we now know you definitely need continuous intakes of certain of the chemicals found in fats. In fact, they're regarded as essential. Animal fats, the fat around a hunk of beef or pork, for instance, are actually the *least important* fats in your diet. Of infinitely more value and importance are the so-called *poly-unsaturated vegetable fats*. We would none of us suffer one iota were all the butter eliminated from our diets entirely. We would all be far better off for it. Butter, as well as the animal fats, are high in saturated fats. It is the saturated fats that, in too high a quantity, cause the fatty deposits which lead to the calcification that causes the plugging up of small and medium-sized arteries. And it is this plugging-up, remember, that is the seat of the trouble in heart disease and strokes, to mention just two diseases that are very common among us today.

So, to sum up on fats, avoid 90 per cent of the fat you find on meat, and switch to vegetable fats to use both as your spread (on bread and toast), and in all your cooking and baking, and forget cream. This way, you'll be getting the essential fats your body needs, *and you'll be preventing in every way humanly possible a later life of artery disease*. Remember, that the poly-unsaturated fats *do not cause fatty deposits in your arteries*.

VITAMINS AND MINERALS. It's quite true, under normal circumstances, that if you are eating a properly balanced diet every day, you don't need extra vitamins and minerals. These vital substances are found naturally in the foods you eat, though in varying quantities. Most people don't utilize these vitamins and minerals in their cooking habits, I'm afraid.

Vitamins and minerals are highest in fruits and vegetables. When vegetables are cooked, most people forget that many of the vitamins and minerals are dissolved in the juice that is left in the pan. Learn to use this vegetable juice as a substitute for gravy on potatoes and bread, or just drink it as part of your meal or as a snack (the juices can be saved by refrigerating them following cooking).

The highest concentration of minerals and vitamins in fruit is located in the white fibrous material just beneath the rind. Don't waste this valuable source of essential vitamins and minerals—learn to snack fruit rind or to grind rinds in making juices. Start eating more potato peel than potato—you'll be getting more vitamins and minerals and less carbohydrate.

The old rule of thumb still applies on vegetables eaten at meals: At least one green and one yellow vegetable at least once a day. This might be corn and green beans, or squash and peas, but both the yellow and the green variety will amply furnish you with the vitamins and minerals you need. And vegetables don't have many calories at all!

Fruit, however, does contain carbohydrate in the form of fruit sugars. Nevertheless, at least one portion of fresh fruit or its canned juice is a necessary part of your daily diet. Canned fruit is permitted, but you should make the habit of buying *water packed* fruit if you use canned fruit—this reduces the carbohydrates since the syrup in food is pure sugar!

If you have reason to suspect you're being shorted on vitamins and minerals, any good general multi-vitamin and mineral preparation can be taken to insure your adequate dietary balance. Vitamins certainly can't hurt you any, but if you have a generous intake of them in your usual diet, remember, your body can't store vitamins for future use. If you have plenty of them in your system at the time, any vitamins or minerals taken in excess will simply be eliminated through your kidneys and bowel.

GAINING THE PROPER BLEND OF COFFEE, TOBACCO AND ALCOHOL

You know, you really don't have to be a purist or a saint to achieve adequate blood sugar control. I've heard many a diet and nutrition expert sternly admonishing their patients not to do this or never to drink that, but I've always wondered if they weren't injecting some of their own prejudices. Smoking, drinking, and the use of coffee are alternately rejected flatly, berated thoroughly, or grudgingly accepted with grave reservations in a variety of ills, and even just on general principles. I, personally, have nothing against liquor, cigarettes or coffee as long as you understand their effects on your blood sugar and are willing to accept moderation as a guide in the use of all three. Consider the following as to their effect in your routine:

COFFEE. Caffeine, the stimulant in coffee, is a safe and reasonable "pick-me-up," especially in the mornings. It is certainly better than the benzedrine group of stimulants we discussed earlier. But, like all stimulants, caffeine taken on an empty stomach *drives down your blood sugar rather rapidly*. To offset this effect, remember that adding skimmed milk to coffee or drinking a glass of skim milk right after coffee will smooth it down. Another way to avoid the lowered blood sugar with coffee is always to eat a snack with it, especially if you like coffee between meals. Coffee taken during meals seldom gives this blood sugar lowering effect unless you drink three or four cups of strong black coffee. This is more than you need; half this amount will suffice. Limit your total intake of coffee to four or five cups a day, and always cover black coffee with a snack. The same rule also applies to tea, cocoa and the cola drinks.

CIGARETTES. These tubes of tars and nicotine are currently the hottest debated subject in the medical profession insofar as their effect on your health is concerned. In my opinion, the key to cigarette smoking is the *number you smoke every day*. A half a pack a day is probably the maximum you can smoke without noticing some ill effects. Five cigarettes a day is even better. Switching to a pipe or cigars is a reasonably safe substitute. The tars and nicotine in cigarettes have a dampening effect on the part of your nervous system that is concerned with the activity of your gastric and intestinal tract. This dampening allows the other half of your nervous system to overstimulate your adrenal glands, thence, your pancreas to produce more insulin. Truly, *the nervous smoker has very poor control of his blood sugar levels*.

As far as all the other anti-health effects of smoking are concerned, I believe they will not be a problem once people learn moderation in their smoking, as well as with many other things that do no harm in small quantities, but become dangerous with overuse. Hardly anything one does in his life escapes this rule of thumb, and smoking is no exception.

LIQUOR. There is no better tranquilizer made by modern pharmacologists than a shot or two of whiskey or gin or a glass of sherry wine. Beyond this amount—a shot or two I mean—a horse of a different color emerges, just as in the case of smoking. The trouble with alcohol is that it's so easy to let the stupor that follows its excess solve one's problems of daily living. Actually, of course, the problems aren't solved at all, but get vastly more complicated in direct proportion to the amounts of alcohol consumed. But alcohol gets people out of contact with their immediate problems—this escape is what seems to many people to be the only answer.

In addition, alcohol eventually has quite serious effects on your health if taken in heavy quantities over a long period of time. Your liver, for instance, can be damaged with far-reaching effects on blood sugar control, as well as on other vital metabolic processes.

The best time for alcohol is at the end of the day, perhaps before dinner, in just enough quantity to bring on a "glow" of relaxation, or just before you're ready to go to bed (always *after* exercising) in just enough quantity to ease the tension, and no more.

DIETING AND EXERCISE INSEPARABLE

Before moving to the next chapter, I'd like to make an important point—one that is often forgotten by people who are overweight or underweight. The point is this: *Dieting and exercise go hand in hand. You can't do an efficient job with either alone.*

Because both your physique and your nutrition are vital keystones to blood sugar control, I can't emphasize the point enough that trying to exercise without also proper dieting, or to diet without properly toning up your muscles is like trying to get dressed without touching your clothes—it can't be done!

Don't even think diet without also thinking exercise, and vice versa.

SUMMARY

1. In order to reverse negative metabolism, you must bring your weight into conformity with your height and frame. Overweight conditions are the most vital to work with, and for every one individual underweight, there are 1,000 who are overweight.
2. Dieting for an overweight condition is really easy: Follow the five rules to the letter and you will succeed admirably. If you are underweight, you don't have nearly the serious problem of your overweight friends, and correcting this is essentially the reverse of the five rules of reducing.
3. Since you cannot hope to begin to control low blood sugar levels and gain vital and lasting good health without weight control, this must be accomplished first, or better, along with proper physical conditioning of your muscles.
4. Appetite control, nutrition and the process of aging influence dieting success. Working at these controls without much regard for your present station in life will insure you a longer life of sparkling health.
5. Dieting and exercise go hand in hand. You can't talk about one without also taking the other into equal account.

4

How to Turn Your Body into a Dynamo of Blood Sugar Energy and Regain Your Youthful Go-Power

In this chapter, I'm going to discuss the second of the keystones of blood sugar control—physical conditioning. I want you to think of this subject as your next goal, now that you've decided to get your weight where it should be for your height and frame.

In this day and age, we find ourselves bombarded by invitations to join health clubs or to try various gimmicks and gadgetry, each supposed to be the last and final answer to "the body beautiful." The trick is that these "new methods" all seem to cost a pile of money. And results depend on maintaining the special schemes for an indefinite length of time—usually until your cash runs out. Wouldn't it be better if you could accomplish complete physical conditioning right in your own home, without having to purchase even the smallest gimmick? How would you like to start feeling the best ever since childhood with only a modest investment of 40–60 minutes each day? I'm going to show you how to do it. All you have to do is follow directions. *And stick with them!*

I'll guarantee this much: If you'll only agree to follow *one* of the various routines suggested in this section, and if you've also started on dietary control of blood sugar, you'll feel so much better physically and be so much more alert mentally, that you won't want to quit!

I want you to view both physical conditioning and diet as *lifelong endeavors* that will keep you on the right track to continual blood sugar control, and as a means to your fullest mental expectations and excellent health during later years.

If I seem to dwell at times on what happens to you in your later years, it's quite intentional. I couldn't possibly recount to you the abject misery, the agonizing weeks and months of pain and debility, or the tragic waste and loss of creative human mind that result from poor habits of blood sugar control during early and middle life. You really don't have to go far to see this, or at least a general idea of it.

Next time you're in a physician's office building, take a close look at the crippled, the debilitated and the infirm who are barely able to get around. Next time you're in a hospital, take a good look in the rooms—notice the people occupying beds who aren't much past their middle years, but who have lost this prime through nothing more than neglect. At your convenience, visit a mental institution or nursing home, take a good look at what happens to body and mind when they are not properly attended. Is this what you want? I don't think so. Vow, today, that you'll strive to gain *complete control of your blood sugar*. Avoid these "last hope" havens of the hopelessly incurable!

THE ROLE OF MUSCLES IN BLOOD SUGAR CONTROL

Remember Jane W. in the first chapter? She was the one who was the "runt"—the congenital weakling of her family. She was brought up to believe this, and believe it she did! She was literally talked into being a poor physical specimen. She'd lived 30 years bearing this cross, but overcame it in three months and surpassed even her wildest hopes within six months! So can you, whether you're 16, 46, 76, or however old!

Take a close look at your physique again. Now that you're doing something about that flab, isn't it sensible to firm up those sagging muscles at the same time? Of course it is. You've already learned that your muscles pile up unimaginable amounts of waste when they are out of shape. Forcing your muscles to work eliminates this waste. Exercising also stimulates blood sugar turnover, helping to control low blood sugar levels by forcing your liver to release stores of vital glycogen and forcing your system to burn up excess stored fat as energy. Think of the vast improvement you'll make in your body by dieting and exercising at the same time!

So important is conditioning to proper blood sugar levels, that I've called *good physical tone the automatic thermostat of low blood sugar control.* Not only does vigorous muscle activity regulate the ebb and flow of blood sugar, but if they're in good condition, muscles exert a feedback effect to the nerve cells in your brain that control them. This feedback works like this:

1. Muscle exercised—waste eliminated from individual cells.
2. Sugar stores stimulated and delivered to these cells.
3. Metabolism becomes positive and dynamic inside cells again.
4. Nerve endings at cell's edges stimulated by this new dynamism.
5. Stimulation travels through nerve in reverse flow of usual direction.
6. Brain cells receive this stimulation and are, themselves, stimulated to vital positive metabolism.
7. As brain cells grow metabolically, they exert more efficient control through nerves to muscle cells—muscle tone increases. And so on, the process being self-perpetuating.

I've heard any number of people in various fields proclaim that man no longer need concern himself with his muscles since his brain—his mind—rapidly is making his muscles obsolete. I can only feel sorry for these people! They're missing the boat completely. Little do they realize that to neglect muscles is also to neglect mind! I admit this much is true: We are, indeed, outstripping our *uses* for muscle power. But that doesn't lower their importance—there isn't one whit of evidence I've seen that Nature is doing away with human muscle tissue as no longer useful or needed, and I've seen plenty of evidence that man, if he keeps up his neglect of physical conditioning, will eliminate himself from the evolutionary march, his mind notwithstanding this trend!

WHAT TO DO ABOUT YOUR CHEST AND ABDOMEN

If you don't start with the same anatomy, you won't, and shouldn't expect to end up looking like Hercules or Venus. It won't happen. But let's do *something* about that chest and that abdomen!

YOUR CHEST. At base, your chest contour is determined by the size and contour of your rib cage and the size of your shoulder blades. You can't change the size or the shape of bones, once they've matured. But you can change the size and shape of the muscles that line the outside of rib cages and shoulder blades. There is nothing like the *push-up* for doing justice to your pectoral muscles, those big ones in front of your chest behind the nipples, and your deltoid muscles, the main part of your shoulders. Push-ups also give you a bonus in doing an excellent job of toning the main arm muscles on the back side of your arms, the triceps, the ones that usually sag down from your upper arm when you extend your arms and hands with palms turned upward.

How to Do Push-ups

To do a push-up, lie flat on the floor on your stomach. Both hands, palms down, on the floor—roughly in line with your shoulders. Now, *make* your arms, chest and shoulders push your body up and off the floor until your arms are completely extended, keeping your legs and stomach absolutely stiff all the while. Once you're up as far as you can push, allow your arms, shoulders and chest muscles to let you down again, but don't quite touch the floor with your stomach or face—just barely above the surface will do. This up-down swing is one complete push-up.

Repeat this up-down cycle until you can't possibly do another one. Let's say you can do ten on first try (don't be at all discouraged if you only do three—they're not easy and you're out of shape, remember). Set your goal at doing 12 or 15 within the next six weeks. You can accomplish this by forcing one more every few days. You'll find that just daily repeating your original ten will develop strength you didn't know you had—first thing you know, you'll be doing an extra one, then another and another. This should be the pattern for all the exercises discussed in this section. Never be discouraged, and certainly not foolhardy, in straining yourself beyond what you feel you can reasonably do with exercise of any kind.

I will personally vouch that when you get to where you can do 30 push-ups in rapid-fire order, without quivering or letting your stomach or legs sag, you won't have the problem of flab on your chest or on the backs of your arms. Push-ups also develop strength in your shoulder blades.

There is a myth floating about some circles, you've heard it possibly, that push-ups aren't good for women to do. Ridiculous! They're harder for women to do, to be sure, because typically women haven't as large pectorals, deltoids and triceps as most men. But you women can and should learn to do them—your improved bust line will show results!

Heart pounding? Huffing and puffing? Good! That's the proof that you did some good with your push-ups. Better rest a minute before going to the next group of sit-ups as follows below.

YOUR ABDOMEN. No one yet has come up with a better toner for your abdomen than the *sit-up*. Sit-ups are also done on the floor, but on your back this time. Begin with your hands clasped behind your neck, and your legs straight out and together. Now, *make your stomach muscles* pull you up to a full sitting position. Touch left elbow to right knee this time, return to the flat position on the floor and next time, touch right elbow to left knee. No fair bending your legs or dropping your hands from their clasped positions. Keep sitting up by using your stomach muscles until they simply won't pull you up another time. Let's say you can do ten the first time. Or is it five? No matter—set your goal for doing twenty in six weeks' time. Use the same technique as with push-ups—add one more every few days. Your stomach muscles are bigger and stronger than your chest and shoulders, so you'll progress faster with these, even though you may feel like someone kicked you in your midsection after the first few days.

When you begin to feel a little self-satisfied with your sit-ups, see if you can rip off about thirty of them in as many seconds. This should take you down a peg or two. But when you can do this, your abdomen will no longer protrude over your belt or through your dress when you stand up, and it will stay slim and trim. You women will find this exercise good for that female "pot" that develops at about 35 years.

Both sexes will find their bowels moving more easily and more regularly as well!

SHAPING UP YOUR ARMS AND LEGS

ARMS. We've already talked about the effect of push-ups on your triceps muscles—the ones, remember, that form the bulk of the back of your upper arm. Now let's look at the muscles in *front* of your upper arm and the ones in your forearms.

The biceps muscle is the one that flexes your forearm—the one the "he-men" are always showing on the front covers of physical culture magazines. It's not necessary to strive for biceps muscles like these pictures. In fact, it is a liability to develop such huge masses of muscle tissue because to keep them that way requires exercising most of the day. Without such constant attention, large, overdeveloped muscles become surrounded by unwanted flab or become "muscle-bound," a condition in which so much effort has been put into muscle development that they are in a constant state of stiffened contraction and practically useless!

The best exercise for your biceps is the "chin-up." This exercise is performed by grasping an overhead pipe or bar with both hands, letting yourself dangle, feet off the ground. Make your arms pull you up to within chin level of the pipe or bar, then let yourself down again. No cheating by letting your feet touch the floor. When you begin chin-ups it's easier to grasp the pipe or bar with the palms of your hands turned toward you. Later, as you progress, turn your palms away as you grasp the pipe—you'll find this position somewhat harder.

The overhead pipe for chin-ups can usually be found around the house—a water pipe in the basement (*not* the hot water pipe!) is usually at hand. In the absence of such a pipe, you can accomplish the same effect by the following method in which the only requirement is any one of the several doorways in your house. With the door open, approach the wall side of the door frame. Stand back away from it, with your left hand fully extended against the frame. Now grab the frame from the other side with your right hand and make your right arm pull you toward the door frame against the resistance of your left arm. For the left biceps, simply do the same thing on the other side of the door frame, pulling against the resistance of your extended right arm. Always keep in mind that if you're right handed, your left side will be the weaker—don't neglect your weak side even though it's harder to accomplish the exercises with it. Make your weak side go through the same motions exactly as many times as your strong side!

FOREARMS. Notice the way your forearm moves when you wind an alarm clock or use a screw driver? This same motion is good exercise for the large muscles of your forearm. Simply grab your right hand, palm down, with your left and grip with your left as hard as you can. Now turn your right palm until it's facing upward against the resistance of the grip of your left hand. Now reverse this motion, and repeat several times. You can accomplish the same effect by doing the palm up, then down, motion while holding a weight in the hand of the arm being exercised. An ordinary iron will do, or even a heavy cast-iron skillet from the kitchen. All forearm movement for this exercise should occur only at the elbow joint.

LEGS. The largest muscles of your body are located in your legs. Treat them well, for they are the ones that allow you to get around. The muscle group in front of your thighs are the quadriceps. They stabilize your knee when you're standing and carry your thigh forward when you walk. Interestingly, they are the first to weaken when you don't use them. The easiest way, of course, to exercise these muscles is to do lots of walking and jogging. Riding a bike is excellent exercise for your legs. Taking stairs instead of elevators should be the rule. Additional tone is given your quadriceps by the squat-stand exercise. This is done by clasping your hands behind your neck, keeping your back straight and squatting down as far as your legs will bend, then *make your legs* stand you back up straight again. This is repeated as many times as you can. When you feel the tone coming back into your legs, hold additional weight in your hands while doing the squats, such as a ten pound bag of flour or sugar or two such weights. This will give stamina to your legs.

The muscles in back of your thighs are the hamstrings, so called because their tendons form thick cords at the back of your knee joint near their attachment. These muscles pull your thigh backwards and are the ones that bend your lower legs. Walking, riding a bicycle, and swimming nicely restore tone to your hamstrings. You can also exercise them by sitting on the floor, pressing the back of your left heel with your right foot, keeping your left leg straight. Now pull back with your left leg against the resistance of your right foot, bending your left leg at the knee joint. Repeat this several times on both sides.

I've mentioned walking and cycling several times in this section. They are two of the best general exercises and conditioners you can do. At least part of your walking or bike-riding should be done in the early morning hours before breakfast. The distance needn't be great at first—a couple of blocks at a fairly brisk pace is sufficient. You can slowly increase the distance until you're walking and cycling at least a mile a day in addition to other exercises you may do during the day. An additional mile can be slowly added in the evenings about two hours following suppertime.

Walking and riding a bicycle not only tone up your legs, increase your breathing and circulation and pep you up in general, but they serve another purpose as well, and this principle applies to all exercise. *Whenever you force a muscle to do extra work, you stimulate new blood vessels to form inside them.* Think what this means! In your heart muscle, the formation of new blood vessels means a stronger, more durable heart that can fight off the occurrence of coronary disease, as well as enable you to recover more efficiently if coronary disease should develop. Your exercise routine may spell the difference between recovery or death in the event of a heart attack!

In your leg muscles, the formation of new blood channels from exercise means less crippling in later life from arthritis and hardened arteries that cause painful disabling leg spasms. These new blood channels mean more efficient blood sugar control, and this means a more vigorous, healthy body and mind!

Start your twice a day program of physical activity today. You'll live to be glad you did!

THE NEGLECTED SMALLER MUSCLES

THE FACE. If you suffer from "the multiple chin," here's what to do to get rid of them. Drop your head downward so your chin touches the upper part of your breast bone, then tighten up the muscles in front of your neck by pulling down and grimacing (smiling broadly) at the same time. With your front neck muscles set in this position, slowly pull your chin up and away from your upper chest until your neck is pulled as far back as you can get it with your chin pointed upward as far as it will go. Feel that area below your jaw strain? That's exactly the idea—stretch your chin as tightly as possible for a few seconds, then repeat the exercise several times. Those multiple chins will soon disappear!

The muscles of your face probably get little, if any, exercise at all. But they need far more attention than this if you're to stay young-looking. Start with your mouth—pucker it out as far as you can get it, then draw it up into an exaggerated smile as tightly as you can. Open your jaws as far as they'll go, then clamp them down as tightly as possible. Repeat these "monkey" grimaces many times. Next, turn down your lower lip, then turn up your upper lip as far as you can. Balloon out your cheeks with your mouth closed. Follow this by sucking in your cheeks with your mouth closed so that your mouth looks like a fish. Then close your eyes as tightly as possible—keep squeezing them closed and at the same time alternate scowling and smiling with your mouth muscles—there's nothing like this for unpacking those bags beneath your eyes!

Scowl, and then look surprised, with your forehead muscles by alternately raising and lowering your eyebrows. This will keep those crow's-feet from aging your face. Next, make your eye muscles move your eyeballs rapidly in every conceivable direction —up, down, sideways, etc. This will keep your six sets of eye muscles toned up.

In short, stretch and contract as forcibly as possible every muscle in your face several times each day. You'll find a mirror helpful in all of these facial exercises (except those in which your eyes are closed), and you can depend on the response of a second party to tell whether you're getting the most from these exercises: If he laughs at your "odd expressions," you're doing them correctly. Toning up facial muscles reduces the fat pads deposited on your face and helps to make your face appear leaner and younger looking. Good facial tone also gives you a much wider range of expressing your emotions—of communicating your feelings to others under a variety of circumstances. Practice face exercises diligently. They will soon pay dividends!

THE NECK. If you seem to be plagued by headaches that start in your neck and gradually spread up the back of your head to include the top and finally, the front of your head, you'll find this exercise helpful, if not curative. First, drop your chin down to the upper part of your breast bone. Then clasp your hands behind your head, and force backward, using only your neck muscles, against the resistance of your clasped hands. Repeat this cycle several times when you feel a tension headache coming on, and routinely at least three times a week. Next, place your right hand against your right temple with your neck bent as far to the left as you can, left ear touching left shoulder. Then bend your neck to the right against the resistance of your right hand. Do the same maneuver using the opposite hand and side of your head. Repeat these side neck movements several times. Next, place your right hand at your right cheek with your head and neck rotated to your left side. Then make your neck muscles turn your head to the right against the resistance of your right hand. Reverse the process for your left side. Repeat this head-turning cycle several times. You've not only mastered the technique for toning your neck muscles, but now, you can overcome stressful neck tightening that distresses you with tension headache!

WHAT TO DO FOR A STRONGER BACK

Virtually 90 per cent of all backache can be traced to poorly toned back muscles. The other 10 per cent represent true difficulties such as the so-called ruptured disc or some other defect of the spine. There is a simple way to tell whether your back trouble is in need of attention by a medical expert. If the pain in your back travels down into your buttock, thigh or even to your lower leg, seek advice *before* starting back exercises. Even when disease is present and it's corrected, you'll find that back exercises under your doctor's supervision can be helpful in restoring a strong pain-free back that doesn't hurt every time you move or bend the wrong way. Your back is the most important mechanism you have for maintaining a straight, graceful carriage. And it's probably poorly attended as far as conditioning goes. Let's get with it and make back toning a daily part of your exercise routine!

The first exercise for your back is done in the following manner. Lie flat on the floor on your stomach and bend both knees so that you can grab your ankles with both hands. Now just rock. Rock back and forth, using your toned up abdomen as the rocker, first head to the floor, then rear back using your legs and arms to pull with. Repeat the rocking motions until your back feels sore, then stop. Try to increase the number of rocks by a few each week. When you can keep up this rocker exercise for about 15 minutes without feeling sore, your back will be stronger, straighter, and you'll find it doesn't strain nearly so easily.

An alternative to this toner for the back is to lie perfectly flat on your stomach, hands and arms outstretched, and make your back muscles lift your legs off the floor, keeping them perfectly straight all the while. Alternate each leg, and repeat several times.

Next, stand up straight, legs about 18 inches apart, and hands down at your sides. Bend at the waist downward until you can see an object located behind you, say, a lamp on the table. Now make your back muscles pull you up straight again and bend over backwards until you see this same object. Repeat this several times, trying to increase the number to 20 or 30 over a period of weeks. Maintain this routine for a permanently stronger back.

REMEMBERING YOUR FORGOTTEN MUSCLES

SHOULDERS. There are muscles in your body you didn't know you had. If you've ever fallen down or have been jolted while riding in a car, you know what I mean. Take the muscles that move your shoulders. Besides the deltoid muscle, the one, remember, that forms the bulk of the shoulder and which you're toning up by doing push-ups, there is a group of muscles that move the shoulder blade up and down and from side to side. These can be toned up in the following manner: Lean against a door frame, using only the back of one shoulder to support your weight against the frame. Now make your shoulder bounce you forcibly away from the frame. The thrust is to the rear. For the opposite set of muscles, the ones that move your shoulder forward, just reverse the process. That is, lean the front part of your shoulder against the frame, facing the doorway this time, and make your shoulders bounce you away from the frame again, the thrust being forward this time. Do this with both shoulders several times. Next, lean against a wall or door frame, your arm fully extended (straight), supporting your weight as you lean. Grab your straightened elbow with the opposite hand (your left hand if you are leaning on your right arm) and make your shoulder muscles twist your extended arm against the resistance of your left hand so that your extended arm turns from palm down to palm up position on the wall. Now just reverse the process—grab the same elbow from the other side, and twist from palm up to palm down position against the resistance of your hand. Repeat this several times.

ARMS. There is a large muscle you use only when you are swinging an axe or a sledge hammer or on the down-swing of a golf drive. It attaches to your back and upper arms. To tone this muscle, stand straight with your right arm bent at the elbow and your upper arm elevated to 90 degrees (as if you're showing off your biceps). Place the palm of your left hand underneath the raised elbow joint and force your elbow down hard against the resistance of your left hand. Do this on both sides and repeat several times. If you can feel your back pull, you're doing the exercise correctly.

Hand muscles are most easily exercised by the simple maneuver of repeatedly squeezing a fairly hard rubber ball, or anything that fits well into your hand and which gives in with pressure. This toner also hardens your forearms, since most of the muscles that work your fingers originate in the forearm. The smaller muscles in your hands can be toned by trying to spread out your fingers against the resistance of the grasp of the opposite hand, and by the reverse of this, namely, by trying to hold your fingers spread out while the opposite hand squeezes them together.

HOW TO VARY EXERCISE ROUTINES

You've probably noticed that so far I've mentioned only exercises that involve absolutely no apparatus other than a doorway or a floor or a wall. You can do quite nicely with only these objects at your disposal. What about weights? I've nothing against them at all. If you can invest around $20.00 for a standard set of vinyl covered, sand-filled weights, or around $8.00 for an exercise bar that can be placed between the frame of any door in your house, you'll be able to make your exercise routine more interesting and challenging. Both weights and exercise bar should last a lifetime.

I believe anyone can mix the two types of exercises I've talked about so far with weights or any other apparatus and come up with several different daily routines that will really make you feel like a new person again. The sit-up and push-up type of exercise, for example, are of the type known as *calisthenics,* made famous during World War II when thousands of young men had to be brought into excellent physical shape as rapidly as possible. The exercises in which the pulling and straining is done against the resistance of another of your own muscles are of the type known as *isometrics,* first popularized by Charles Atlas, the familiar muscular man on the back of comic books of a generation ago. Working with weights has both advantages and disadvantages. Remember the following points if you're going to work with weights:

ADVANTAGES
1. Weights build muscle stamina quickly and increase the size of muscles more than other exercises.
2. You don't have to work out quite as long with weights to accomplish strength building in your muscles.
3. If you're a rather strong individual to begin with, weights will challenge you more than calisthenics or isometrics.

4. If you're a slightly built individual to begin with, and are trying to enlarge your muscles, weights will help to do the job more efficiently.

DISADVANTAGES

1. It's easier to strain your muscles with weights than with the other two types of exercises.
2. It's easier to overdo exercises with weights—*do not* attempt to press weight exercises beyond what is obviously your limit until you have spent at least *six months* with weight-lifting.
3. It's easier to become "muscle-bound" with weights. Remember the principle I stated earlier: Always exercise muscles that work in opposition to the ones you're exercising *equally* as much. (If you do ten presses with a 45 pound weight, do also ten curls with the same amount of weight.)
4. You can't exercise as many muscles with weights as you can with calisthenics and isometrics.

With a set of weights, there is usually one long bar with a variety of weights that can be attached to both ends of the bar. There are usually two or three short bar-bells for use with a single hand and arm with smaller weights that attach to the ends. The long bar is to be used with *both* hands. Start low—10–15 pounds on either end—and do the following routines. Remember that *balance is important.*

PRESS. This is done by positioning the long bar behind your head with both hands so that the bar rests on your shoulders and back. Now, make your triceps muscles push up the weight so that it's hoisted into the air, both arms fully extended, then back down again. The press can also be done by lying flat on the floor and holding the bar across your chest—pressing up the weights (the same muscles are used) until both arms are fully extended, then back down again.

CURL. This maneuver is done standing straight with your feet a little apart. Hold the bar across the front of your thighs with both hands, palms turned up. Now, bend up your arms until the bar lies across your chest, then return the bar to its original position. This exercise utilizes your biceps muscles—just the opposite of the press that exercises the triceps.

FLOOR JERK. With the middle of the bar resting on the floor beside your right or left foot, bend over and make your shoulders jerk the weight off the floor until it's at a level with your chest, then back down. Repeat this several times, then do the same using the other side.

SHOULDER CURL. With one of the smaller bars, two and a half to five pounds on either end, hold the weight down at your side with your right hand. Slowly raise your right arm until it's fully extended above your head, then back down. No bending your elbows on this one. Make your deltoids do the work.

ARM WIND. With the smaller bar (carrying five or ten pounds) in your hand, flex your arm to 90 degrees and slowly twist your forearm palm up then palm down. Repeat these twisting movements several times on both sides.

How a 40-Year-Old Man Built Up His Health

A man of 40 years whom I know has developed a good, flexible routine utilizing all three types of exercises. He is five feet ten inches tall and weighs 160 pounds—he's in as good a shape for his age as anyone I've met, and has achieved absolute control over his blood sugar. I'll pass his routine along to you for consideration. Over the past few years this particular man, call him Carl, has shaped his physique to about what it was when he was 17 years old. Before he started, he weighed 180 pounds, was sluggish and lazy, and had about as much stamina as a piece of wet spaghetti. He began by doing sit-ups in the morning on arising. He found he could only do about five without feeling like he'd been hit by a car in his mid-section, but within four months, could easily do 30 in as many seconds. He followed his sit-ups by doing isometrics for his chest and shoulders. This he did by clasping his hands, elbows turned outward, and pressing his hands together for several seconds, then relaxing, then pressing some more. For his chest, he folded his arms in front of his chest and pressed inwardly with both arms, and at the same time squared his shoulders backward. He found this contracted his pectorals much like a push-up would do. He'd then step to a door frame narrow enough so that with both arms flexed at his sides, his elbows touched either side of the frame, then he pushed both elbows toward the sides of the frame, forcing his deltoid (shoulder) muscles to work against the resistance of the door frame. He spent about ten minutes with this routine in the morning. At night, just before retiring, he would do push-ups first. For some time he could do only eight because his arm muscles were small. Within six months, he could easily manage 20 in as many seconds. Next, he used the back-bending exercise I've described, in which you bend over and look at an object between your legs, then bend backwards until you see the same object. He soon was able to do 20 of these rapidly. The last thing he did at night was his facial isometrics as I've described. He soon lost his double chin, his face became lean, and wrinkles and fat over his cheeks disappeared completely.

For variation after about a year of this routine, he began to alternate his morning sit-ups with isometrics for his abdomen. This he did by standing straight and sucking in his stomach as far as he could, following which he made his abdomen muscles contract, bending over at the waist, then repeating this cycle. On other mornings, he would use the scissor-kick to exercise his abdomen. The scissor is done by lying on the floor, flat on your back, hands clasped behind your neck. Both legs are raised about 18 inches off the floor, knees straight at all times, then swinging them out as far as they'll go, then back in again, crossing one leg over the other. On the next swing, the opposite leg is crossed on the inward swing. Carl soon progressed to fifty complete scissors. In another year, he developed the variation of doing sit-ups at the same time he was doing his scissors kicks! This man's waist is as flat and hard as it was in his teens, and believe me, it will stay that way if he keeps doing the sit-ups with the scissor kicks at the same time.

Carl acquired a set of weights not long ago, and every other night he uses these in the manner I described. He doesn't have a flabby muscle in his body, and reports that he hasn't had a day of illness in five years! It's interesting that Carl used to be plagued by two or three episodes of infectious bronchitis every winter. He'd cough and hack up phlegm for at least ten days and end up having to take a course of antibiotic drugs to clear it up. Since he began to take his blood sugar into hand with diet and exercise and has switched to a pipe and only three cigarettes a day, he hasn't had one chest cold! Incidentally, Carl spends 15–20 minutes twice a day with his exercise routine. He maintains his superb physical shape by spending only 30–40 minutes a day, and so can you. Begin now!

HOW TO GIVE YOUR HEART AND LUNGS A HEALTH BREAK

I want to emphasize again the bonus exercising brings. Every cell in your body needs constant and adequate oxygen and sugar to perform at their peak. Every time you strain one of those flabby muscles, you're increasing the supply of both these vital substances to cells all over your body. No matter what your exercise routine, you're making your heart exert a little each time—exert more than it ordinarily would. This heart muscle exertion causes not only new blood vessels to form, thereby furnishing the heart pump with a more efficient *blood sugar supply,* but also forces your heart to start its own protection against injury and disease as well! I don't think Carl, in the case mentioned a bit ago, will ever have a coronary occlusion, but if he should happen to have one, his heart will pull through with flying colors. So will yours if you want to take the few minutes a day to start getting those muscles in shape.

The same applies to your lungs. Those thousands of little air sacs are being stretched, and the muscle layers that surround them are being toned-up with every forced breath your exercising makes you take. This in turn raises their ability to absorb air with its vital oxygen supply. The net result increases the sugar and metabolic turnover in all your tissues, including, remember, those important endocrine glands. Your glands work more efficiently and your mind, in turn, responds with vigor and dynamic activity, leading to better productivity and creativity. How can you lose? Your exercise routine literally makes a new person of you, inside and out!

ADJUSTING YOUR EXERCISE ROUTINES

I've mentioned that on arising and just before retiring at night are the two prime times for your exercise routines. If you want to add a third, by all means do so. Just remember the following points:

1. Exercise *before* mealtime, not afterwards.
2. Take the week-end off, especially, if you're reasonably physically active on Saturdays and Sundays. There's no need to run it into the ground.
3. Take in some extra energy following exercising: a sandwich, a glass of skim milk, a salad or jello. *Not* candy, sugar or baked goods like cookies or cake.
4. If you feel punk for some reason when you're just starting your routine (you won't feel anything but vitally healthy when your routine is well established!), forget the routine until you feel well again. The routine takes adjusting on the part of your body—give it time, you've got the rest of your life before you!
5. If you have a condition that's been there for a while, consult your doctor *before* you get too engrossed in exercise routines—get his blessing if he's treating some physical condition.
6. If you're past 50 years old, healthy and want to stay that way, don't be afraid to start an exercise routine *now*. Just plan on taking more time to build up to things and don't try to imitate the routine of someone half your age.

This question of age has arisen many times. As age progresses, comes a sharpness of mind. This actually helps you to start dieting and exercise routines. And once you start them, you'll feel the youthful vigor returning to your body, and your mind will retain that sharpness and keenness associated with being alert and mature. In fact, if there's a secret to keeping razor-sharp wits and alert incisive minds with the aging process, it's in keeping physically fit so that you retain control over your blood sugar levels. It's as simple as that.

Of course, no one expects you to do at 60 years what you or

anybody else can do at 30 years. This would be silly, as well as impossible. But you can and should keep that body and mind in as good a shape as possible by good habits of diet and exercise. At the end of the book you'll find a section listing alternate exercises for variation. Learn to utilize all of these and even invent new ones for yourself!

SUMMARY

1. Good physical tone is the automatic thermostat for your control of blood sugar. Physical tone and proper diet go hand in hand. Size up your physical condition and promise yourself that you'll start *today* to do something about correcting it.

2. The major groups of muscles in your chest, abdomen and extremities are the easiest to start with in developing your exercise routine. Concentrate on them, using the variety of calisthenics, isometrics and weight lifting routines given in this section.

3. When you've got the feel of exercising these large muscle groups, go to the smaller muscle groups and don't forget your back. To forestall stiff, unyielding disease joints, and to stabilize your back, the center of your upright position, include these muscles in part of your exercise routines every day.

4. The efficient control of blood sugar levels is not only absolutely dependent on good muscle tone and diet habits, but also acts as its own energizer. The better your blood sugar control becomes, the easier it is to exercise and the better your blood sugar control becomes.

5. Good diet and exercise routines done every day, with the exception of week-end breaks and ill-health, carries its own bonus: Your heart, blood vessels and lungs automatically improve their function. This, in turn, automatically improves blood sugar control.

6. Age should present no problem to exercise routines. If you tailor your activity to what you know you can do, and if you keep this up, even if it's not like that of your 30-year-old next door neighbor, you will benefit in both mind and body.

7. Exercise has a reciprocal effect on mind: The better tone the muscles, the better the brain cells perform. Retain a sharp, keen, creative mind by starting your exercise routine today.

5

How to Use Blood Sugar Control
to Energize Your Mind

You have now reached a milestone. You're feeling better than you have in your entire life because you're eating and exercising properly, and you've started to mobilize the vast reservoir of metabolic activity that will bring perfect control of your blood sugar. Perhaps some of you have yet to be convinced that this reservoir can be tapped, or that it even exists. Don't despair! It's your mind that you now need to work with—you need that extra spark, a firm push, to start up the amazing power plant that resides in your body. And where does such a spark—such an inspiration—come from? It comes directly from your own mind!

I'm going to discuss in this chapter what mind really is, what makes it tick, and how you can reach the depths of your own mind to bring forth from its hidden recesses the vital essence that can unlock doors for you that you've never dreamed possible. And with mind control you'll have mastery over blood sugar and continuing vigorous health. I'll discuss conscious, sub-conscious and para-conscious mind, and the connection of these mind parts with thinking and creativity. The subject of ESP and how to train yourself to use it will be covered. And I'll show you how to overcome habits that hold you in their grip, as well as how to resolve forever the nagging business of mental "inferiority" that reflects itself in do-nothingness.

In short, I intend to show you how to use what nature has provided you with in the form of your brain.

WHAT IS MIND?

This question has stumped poets, philosophers and biologists for centuries. Mind is unique in the entire biological system in that man, alone, is the sole possessor of this fabulous tool among creatures. Mind is a bonus, a super-numerary, a special kind of force, if you will, arising as a result of the unique combination of brain and body. Mind *must* be regarded as this country's—any country's—most precious natural resource, second to none! The only remorse about the human mind that I can think of is that such a versatile, profoundly useful and influential power is so seldom used to the fullest advantage of the one who owns it—*you!* People keep talking about what a "fine mind so-and-so has," or wishing they had just "half his brains" in speaking about a particularly sharp individual. It's like wishing you had a uranium mine when you're standing right on top of it—you *do* have every bit as good a mind as any other person. There are people with a special flair for mathematics or with artistic ability or with a special gift for dreaming up mechanical gadgets. But these are *talents,* and every one of us has some talent. Talents have nothing to do with *mind.* Your mind is a special by-product of your brain and your body. It's a tool that nature gave you to use. Mind is one of those items found occasionally that adds up to much more than the sum of all its known parts! All you have to do is decide you're going to put your mind to work.

And how, you may reasonably ask, can something add up to *more* than the total of its parts? Take the example of the train I used earlier. You have an engine and a string of cars hooked together. The engine can move with its own power down the tracks, but it's not a train. The hooked-up cars can't move under their own power, but they can haul freight or passengers (not many of the latter today). But, the hooked-up cars are not a train. Put them together and they form a unique object—a train in its complete sense. Take another example. A piece of metal called sodium is shiny, soft and so unstable in air it has to be stored in kerosene or in a vacuum or it bursts into flame and evaporates away. A greenish gas called chlorine floats through the air and is so irritating and noxious it would poison you if you should happen to breath enough of it. Neither of these elements are compatible with your health. But combine them, and what do you have? Common table salt! A product vastly different from either sodium or chlorine and actually essential to your life processes!

In a similar way, your mind is the unique result of all the parts of your brain *plus* all the parts of your body—*your blood sugar* and hormones, remember, influence your mind—*plus* all the various parts of your environment that are capable of influencing your brain like light, sound, touch, smell, experience and emotions. Put these things together, and you have a mind.

BODY VERSUS MIND

Here is another question that has provoked many an argument. I've heard colleagues discuss the question whether, if the human brain could be removed and preserved, the mind would still function. In view of what is known about mind from the previous discussion, the answer is definitely *no*.

Try as many medical specialists may, including psychiatrists, mind and body cannot, nor is it likely that they ever will, function separately. This precept was recognized by the great physicians of the past, but it has not been made strong enough in today's rush to super-specialization. Any attempt to further carve the human carcass into its component parts and to try to deal with them singly as though they were separate entities will be fraught with the impossible. I'd like you never to think of mind without also thinking of body, nor of body without deliberating its permanent link to mind. They're as inseparable as table salt!

You may recognize a thread of similarity here with some things I've mentioned already—the idea of good muscle tone affecting the cells in the brain, and the principle of will power in starting good practices of blood sugar control, of diet and of exercise. Yes, a smoothly functioning mind and good physical health *do* go together. They *have* to go together! *You can take another step toward blood sugar control by learning how to mold your mind so that it's in step with your body.*

HOW YOUR MIND THINKS AND CREATES

THINKING. Your mind thinks in symbols. The earliest form of communication was also done with symbols, languages having developed because man had to be more precise with all the communicating he found necessary. You can, of course, force written words into your thinking, and perhaps visualize a written page or document by summoning it up from memory, but most thinking is done with symbols, not in languages. There are some who tell us that thinking is just a glorified conditioned reflex: Ring a bell and offer a plate of food enough times, and soon just ringing the bell will make the mouth water, a simple form of a conditioned reflex. Such a notion is only partly true. Almost all thinking involves the past experiences of the thinker. But there's more to it. Thinking also involves the special ability of mind to *project* itself into a variety of situations—to visualize yourself, for instance, right in the middle of a circumstance that hasn't really occurred yet, and to draw conclusions from this "future projection" of yourself into a situation.

Thinking also involves logic, a kind of thinking quite apart from conditioning or projection. Logic means the drawing of conclusions based on known facts about just part of a situation. For instance, if you know that all men are mortals and that Thomas Edison was a man, then you can conclude that Thomas Edison was also a mortal. Thinking also involves the total of your experiences and the emotions that are connected with them. If you once fell off a horse and broke your leg, it's quite likely that any thought concerning horses or broken limbs will have unpleasant emotions of some kind along with it—fright, pain, and so on—because of the special experience unique to your past.

CREATIVITY. When you create something, you turn into a reality what is inside your head—what is at first only a thought. But this thought is different; it's a genuinely new and unusual thought peculiar to you and you alone. It may well have the influence of someone else incorporated in it, but the main part of your creation is pure *you*. How does your mind accomplish this task? Invent something that apparently hasn't existed before? It isn't the mystery that it appears at first glance. Creation on the part of the mind is probably the outcome of a tremendous job of association and integration—that is, from all your experiences, your feelings, your desires, suddenly appears a *mosaic*. A mosaic is a pattern of basic things put together a bit differently, or perhaps quite a bit differently, than you or anyone else has seen or heard before. An example of this would be a person keenly interested in machines of all types and varieties—someone who devotes a lot of time to thinking about gadgetry. He's already familiar with most machines, their parts, and how they fit together to form a whole. Suddenly, he has a flash. He "sees" in his mind's eye a new machine. He makes detailed drawings of his mind "picture," assembles the parts together, and has created a new machine. His mind has shuffled around all the bits and pieces of known machines so many times and so rapidly that from the possible combinations has come a mosaic of a different machine. The same might be true of an author of fiction—from his experiences and from actual research into a certain subject, his mind devises a story from one of many possible combinations of all the facts. He sharpens the plot, gives character to his heroes and villians and has, when finished, created a story.

IS MIND A GLORIFIED COMPUTER?

If someone could or would do it, he would have to build a computer as big as a house and constantly attended by several dozen technicians just to perform the ordinary simple "switchboard functions" of your brain. Your mind does all these switchings, plus a host of other tasks, such as controlling your endocrine glands, plus it thinks and creates, judges and projects, and it *feels* —activities no computer will ever approach! And your mind does this all within the relatively small confines of your skull and on a power expenditure of less than 25 watts—less than it takes to power a single Christmas tree light! Do you really believe a computer will ever match this for sheer economy of effort? Or for sheer magnitude of accomplishment? I don't. When next you hear some misguided soul speak of your brain as about to be put out of business by a computer, pity him—he just doesn't understand the power of his own mind!

WILL POWER AND CONCENTRATION—
THE KEYS TO MIND CONTROL

WILL POWER. Why was a young man I once operated on for a hernia found walking that same afternoon in the hospital lobby, straight and composed, as though nothing had happened? Why didn't he need pain medicine during his post-operative period? Why was another patient I treated able to terminate her migraine headaches within 30 minutes after they started when it usually takes all day—sometimes two or three days—for a migraine attack to stop? How is it that another man I know is able to produce anesthesia at will around any area of his anatomy he chooses, and have teeth pulled or cavities filled without anesthetics of any kind? *Sheer will power.* These people aren't stage performers or charlatans, nor were they trying to impress anyone with tricks—they just did the feats as a matter of course. They have learned the secret of will power and some of the things its mastery can bring. They have learned that understanding the underlying disturbance or cause for some states of ill-health enables them, by determined effort of mind (will power) to alter these states. So can you if you care to learn the knack.

I asked the young man of the first example above whom I attended some years ago what his secret was. "How do you stand up like that so soon after surgery without feeling like a newly strung tennis racket?" I asked him later. He smiled and said it was really simple. "All I did," he said, "was concentrate the night before the operation that I would awaken from the anesthetic without discomfort." I didn't believe a word of it—then. Now, after some years of observing others do essentially the same thing, I accept the explanation as a fact. If only this could be taught to everybody! Surely the suffering in this old world would be far less.

The second case, a middle-aged woman with migraine headaches for some years, told me that once she understood *why* she had the pain, she concentrated on reversing the effect. And it worked! In a migraine attack, the blood vessels in the head go through two stages: They dilate (become enlarged and engorged with blood), then they constrict (clamp down tightly). The first stage is when migraine sufferers have the peculiar feelings, flashing lights, spots in front of their eyes, and sometimes even partial blindness for a short while. When the second stage begins (the constriction), the migraine sufferer gets his severe sledge-hammer headache that sometimes lasts for a day or two and can completely incapacitate him. This patient told me that when I explained to her the reason for the symptoms, she reasoned that if she could prevent the vessels from constricting (the action of the commonly used drugs in migraine), she might get better relief without drugs which aren't usually 100 per cent effective. She was successful! She did it by concentrating during the first stage on making her blood vessels stay dilated.

The man with the ability of spontaneous anesthesia had the same answer. He simply concentrated on numbness in a certain area and it came. He did say that he didn't learn the trick overnight—it took him about two years to perfect his technique. But I've seen a dentist pull a tooth from this man's jaw and he didn't bat an eye!

All three of these people were determined to overcome, and they did. This is will power at work. You can probably already think of a dozen different ways you can begin to use *your* will power.

CONCENTRATION. Notice that the word *concentration* appears more than once in the foregoing cases. To put your will power to work requires *first and foremost* that you learn the art of concentration.

Concentration is best described as the ability to put everything else out of your mind except that on which you want to concentrate. The object of your concentration can be a name, a person, a piece of furniture, a number, or anything you select. Fix your complete and uninterrupted attention on the object, whatever it is. Close your eyes, if it's easier, or keep them wide open—it makes no difference. Just make that one object the subject of your uninterrupted attention. When you find you can do this for five minutes without having other thoughts or being distracted by anything else in your environment, you've mastered concentration.

You may know someone who seems, at times, to be "miles away," although he's right next to you in the same room. You may strike up a conversation with him, but he obviously hears nothing you're saying. Then he "comes back," and is his usually attentive and well-organized self again. He's been concentrating. And he's learned it so well that he can do it any time and anywhere. This is concentration at its best. Learn to copy this habit. When you have a spare five or ten minutes and can relax for awhile, practice concentration. In no time at all, you'll be able to do full concentration, and you'll be ready to use this tool to help with blood sugar control and mind utilization.

CAN AUTOSUGGESTION HELP YOUR MIND?

Now that you understand what concentration is and are well on your way to learning it, you can prove the power of auto-suggestion for yourself with this easy and useful routine. After your evening exercise work-out has been accomplished and you've gone to bed, put everything else out of your mind except the picture of a face of a clock showing the time you want to awaken the next morning Now concentrate on this picture—suppose the clock face shows seven o'clock—and *in your mind* (not aloud) repeat the phrase, " will awaken at seven o'clock." Repeat this phrase 10 or 15 times with nothing else on your mind but the picture of that clock face. Then put the entire matter to rest— forget it, dissolve into the restful sleep that your exercise has induced. You'll be amazed that you will, indeed, awaken at or very near the suggested time! If you should happen to fail the first time, don't be discouraged—just continue it each night until success comes. You'll get the hang of it very soon.

With this easy step you've mastered the essence of autosuggestion! You've taken the first move toward reaching your inner mind and making it work for you! You may now see how the young man was able to enjoy an apparently "miraculous" recovery from ordinarily painful surgery. He did it by autosuggestion, just as you've done by using your built-in alarm clock, except that where you pictured a time on a clock face, he simply substituted the repeated suggestion that he would awaken from the anesthetic without pain! You may now see the middle-aged woman learned to terminate her painful migraine. She did it by autosuggestion as you have done, except that she substituted a picture of a blood vessel in a dilated (relaxed) state and repeated to herself that her head blood vessels would remain in that state. The same applies to the man who could numb his teeth—he mastered the art of autosuggestion so well that he could block-off specific areas of his body and not feel pain in them.

Do you now see other possibilities? *Some exciting new ways to gain control of blood sugar through mind control?* What about some of those nagging symptoms listed in Chapter 2? Might you not now have another tool to use to overcome them? Or how about your diet? Having a hard time with your appetite? Use autosuggestion to discipline yourself—use it also to overcome those aches and pains that go with straining soft muscles. Use autosuggestion to make your mind create and to think more clearly.

HOW CONSCIOUS AND SUB-CONSCIOUS MIND WORK FOR YOU

CONSCIOUS MIND. Conscious mind is that part of your thinking and mental activity that continues while you are awake and alert. It's the *aware* part of your being—the part that tells you where you are, what you're doing, and what to do next.

Parts of your conscious mind include judgment, decision-making, calculating with figures, your five senses of seeing, hearing, touching, smelling, testing, and all the things that go into moving about in the environment in which you live and work. It's your conscious mind, for instance, that tells you it's time to do your exercises when you first climb out of bed. It is your conscious mind that accepts or rejects the idea of your dieting. Your conscious mind is at this very moment wrestling with the words and meanings that this page is imprinting upon it. Your conscious mind may be saying to you that this stuff you are reading is all hogwash— I hope it isn't, but some conscious minds are quite skeptical. There is a part of your conscious mind, however, that deals with fair play and a sense of good sportsmanship. If your mind finds the material in this section hard to swallow to this point, please allow the fair play of it to at least give the material a chance to soak in, and to at least *try* some of the suggestions offered thus far. You may find that your conscious skepticism is modified and changed a little. If it is, then the book will have been worthwhile.

Conscious mind is the realistic part of your constitution. You'd be surprised if you knew how much information your brain picks up every minute of your waking hours, yet filters out before allowing it to reach your thinking. One of conscious mind's duties, as a matter of fact, is to reduce the burden of things you have to remember and think about while you're awake. Sometimes, the filter is too efficient—and a habit of thinking forms in your mind that shuts out important things you *should* think of more often. At other times, the filter is not efficient enough and your mind is flooded with many things that aren't very important to your well-being. If this happens at night, you have a hard time getting to sleep—you have insomnia. What is it that keeps this filter working up to snuff? Yes, it's your blood sugar levels, of course. It may not seem strange to you now to see the connection of your entire outlook on life, should your blood sugar levels be too low —*your conscious mind simply can't do a proper job without efficient and constant levels of blood sugar!*

SUB-CONSCIOUS MIND. Your sub-conscious mind is the "receiving dock." Everything you do, everything that happens to you, and all your feelings are recorded by your sub-conscious mind. All of it is carefully stored. Thousands of people have been regressed under hypnosis to recall events and to summon emotional responses to situations that happened in their childhood. I'm familiar with a group of patients who, under the hypnotic guidance of a psychiatrist, were actually able to recall events during the first minutes of their birth!

If this is true, why do you have such a time trying to recall all those things that seem to slip your mind? Because your sub-conscious activity, remember, is supervised by your conscious mind— a lot of what your sub-consicous mind records is filtered out. If this were not the case, your thinking mind would be so cluttered with minutia and detail that you wouldn't get anything else done during the day except think about all the things that have composed your life up to now! But the information is there, nonetheless. You can train your sub-conscious to recall events and persons, places and things, and most anything else you wish by utilizing autosuggestion in the same manner as you use it to awaken you in the morning. Simply concentrate on the event or thing you want to remember, and it will come. Sometimes the information asked for will be a day or two in coming. Sometimes, you'll awaken in the middle of the night with the requested material shining forth like a light.

Your sub-conscious mind is the reservoir of other talents as well. It is the storehouse of your reflexes, the things you do "unconsciously" having made the response repeatedly. Your protective mechanisms are part of this area of your mind. A loud noise is made, and you reflexly jump, duck or look toward the direction of the noise. You touch something hot, and you reflexly draw your hand or fingers away from the heat source. Your sub-conscious is always trying to keep you out of trouble. Your subconscious acts as repository for all those things your conscious mind may reject even though such things may be logically a part of conscious mind. For example, you may have received a serious injury as a child through an auto accident or from being kicked by a horse. The feelings attached with the event of this accident may have been so strong that your conscious mind may have chosen to "bury" the memory and feelings connected with it to protect you from going through discomfort by having to think about it over and over again. The trouble with such buried material is that it has a habit of cropping up again, sometimes much later in life, this time, in a disguised form such as a fear of automobiles or a loathing of horses. One method used in psychiatry, as a matter of fact, consists of going over such earlier occurrences and reacting again to the incident, this time in a more mature, "understanding" fashion.

WHAT IS SPIRIT?

The human spirit may be said to represent the zest for living—the energizing power for life, in other words. If a person has given up hope, has become disenchanted with everything and everybody around him, and feels there's really no use or purpose in his or in anyone else's life, his spirit is said to be broken. I think it's best that the word spirit be reserved in this way and not tied to a religious meaning for reasons I'll discuss later. At any rate, the human spirit is what makes men rise to new heights of achievement, development and virtue. *Spirit is what you are lifting when you gain control of your blood sugar levels and begin to live life with purpose and direction instead of drudgery and self-pity.*

What has spirit to do with mind? In order to bring mind to its highest perfection and potential, you must have that charge of electricity that says to you inside, "I'm *going* to do it. I *will* do it." If this charge does not come, your efforts will be in vain. This is why, for instance, you must start with diet and exercise to control blood sugar: The control of body brings on control of mind because the two are interconnected and inseparable. You could start in the reverse fashion, that is, bring about body control starting with mind. But I've found this approach much more difficult and harder to do. Therefore, I think you have done the correct and the most efficient job by first conditioning *your body, then your mind*.

THE FANTASTIC SCOPE OF YOUR MIND

Did you ever stop to think what your mind really means? How wide the horizon of its influence? Consider the following.

PHILOSOPHY. Philosophy is the mother knowledge. You and I live our lives under the principles of certain philosophies whether we realize it or not. Sometimes, our philosophies change, sometimes not. We all *do* philosophy every day in our lives. If you believe in the principle, "me first, everybody else second," then you subscribe to one philosophy concerning human relationships. If you believe the Universe was created by someone with man-like qualities, that's one religious philosophy. If you believe that Communism is a constant threat and needs to be wiped out at all costs, this is one political philosophy. If you believe Communism is a flash in the pan and vastly over-rated as a world threat, this is yet another. So you may begin to see that you don't have to be in an armchair puffing on a pipe to practice philosophy —you practice it all the time! The point is this: The mind is what puts philosophies together. Minds conceive and practice philosophies. Your mind, then, is one of many that gives the world its many bodies of basic principles from which virtually all activity, all opinion, and all goals are formed!

SCIENCE AND THE ARTS. That all technology is based on the advancement of science is no mystery. Without scientific endeavor, there would be no automobile, no jet planes, no wash and wear fabrics, and no computers. The science of physics, for example, would still be little more than a curiosity without the minds of people like Newton, Maxwell and Einstein. Scientific technical advance depends absolutely on the minds of thousands of people who devote their lives and their minds to this work.

In the field of music, where but from the minds of a Beethoven, a Gershwin or a Rodgers and Hammerstein could such treasures emerge? How could we ever measure the contribution of Rembrandt or daVinci? Or our great literary works? All great men and women of science and the arts have one thing in common, if little else: Their *minds* have given to all of us a more pleasant world in which to live. Is this not mind control at its finest?

LOVE. One of the greatest of human virtues and one of the least commonly seen these days is love. Besides being a virtue, love is also an emotion—a feeling—one has for another. Where do emotions reside? In the mind. I've seen a good many definitions of love. Some by poets of renown, others by ministers and philosophers, and still others by psychoanalysts. All are well worthwhile, but I believe if one has to have a quality like love defined for him, his mind isn't all it should be. If you don't have a very special feeling for others, especially those close to you, that tells you that this feeling *is* love without actually being able to describe or define it, then you're in trouble. I see a good many people who probably never experience love in any form. These people haven't known what it is to love *themselves* as yet, and this is the reason they can't find room in their lives for love of others. Other people finally learn to love themselves, but with this they are stuck. They love *only* themselves and find no reason to share such an emotion with another. Those for whom it can be honestly said that they have learned to love others equally as well as themselves have always been a rare breed and are becoming rarer. This is sad, for no mind can really reach its zenith without love.

I mention these few areas: Philosophy, Science and the Arts, and Love to show you in what wide application your mind must work. In what great complexity mind must function! Start today enlarging the horizons of your mind!

HOW TO CONTROL YOUR MIND IN A TROUBLED WORLD

Although I don't think the drug-taking habit which has been "in" during the past two years represents the leaning of a majority of young people today, I think it does represent an underlying problem rampant not only in youth, but also in older people, many of whom are these drug-taking youngsters' parents. This problem is the lack of mental discipline. The case of a young man of 20 I met about two years ago is an example of what I mean. The fact that he happened to be taking acid, hippie slang for LSD, doesn't alter the fact of his trouble or that of his parents.

Case History of a "Hippy"

As with many hippies, Pat came from an excellent home. His father was a physician, and his mother a devoted and well-motivated homemaker. He had one younger brother. Pat was in his freshman year at college just three months when he began to lose control of his good sense—he took his first LSD trip. Then followed more. Pat couldn't remember just how many. He quit school. He became sloppy in dress, manner and personal hygiene. He slipped into atrocious habits of eating and got practically no exercise at all. And he started sleeping with a number of young girl hippies to show his "love for all mankind."

When his parents, worried sick because they didn't know where Pat was living, or if he was, finally located him and brought him home, he was drugged to the point of lunacy. For this reason, Pat's parents reluctantly admitted him to a mental hospital, and this is where I first got to know him. What pushed him into such a life when he had so much going for him—an interested well-to-do family, a chance for an excellent education that could take him as far as he wished, and a good mind? Pat's first answer was from the stock I've heard so many times from kids in his predicament: "Man, I wanted to turn on—live, man, live!" I knew Pat had more brains than this, so I told him I thought he was lying, and I wanted a straight answer, right now! This kind of surprised him. When he recovered, he began to pour out a story that included the following hard facts:

1. He'd never really understood what "he" was—his self-image seemed never to materialize as he grew up.
2. No one at home really set goals for Pat to reach—his father occasionally alluded to the idea of medicine as a career, and seemed to think Pat would take this for granted. No one ever bothered to ask Pat what was on his mind.
3. Pat's folks had given him almost everything he wanted— as a youth, every whim was satisfied, every demand met, and then some. He'd never wanted for anything. And nothing was ever demanded in return—if he wanted to work, fine; if not, that was fine, too.
4. Pat said that he just got tired of double standards in the home. He was tired of hearing his folks preach one thing and turn right around and either do or say the opposite when the circumstances warranted. He said the same thing about college and society at large. He said that to him, national politics is the biggest joke he'd ever heard of and that our conduct in foreign affairs is a national scandal.

Now whether Pat was right or wrong in his appraisal of the situation, this was the way he saw it. This is how it looked through his eyes. There must be a good deal of food for thought in what he told me for our social experts to study. What Pat was actually doing, of course, was "turning himself off" with LSD, not "turning on," as the phrase goes.

I watched Pat get well, and I saw him leave the mental institution, having freed himself from the need for drugs, having established good habits of physical conditioning and having gained back the 30 pounds he'd lost while on his drug bender. He had control of his mind again. He returned to college and is doing well to this day. I must say that he is a changed young man. He has overcome the first three of the four parts of what he saw as his problem. He is determined to do something "personally," as he put it to me later, about the fourth item. And I hope he succeeds! He realized, you see, that it does little good to "drop out and turn on" (to use drugs). The problems, deep-seated and disgusting though they may be, remain. Such problems must be solved, and getting control of his good mind and training it *to do something* about what he considered important issues of the day, was the first order of business. It's a lot like what I talked about earlier in this section about the conscious mind's tendency to "bury" some of life's more agonizing experiences. The fact that they're out of mind doesn't mean that they're solved or safely tucked away forever—they have the habit, remember, of jumping up again, perhaps in a disguised form, but present, nevertheless.

You can profit from Pat's experience even though you probably don't take drugs like he did. You are *you*—an individual of unique and special characteristics. It's *you* who must set goals and strive toward them. It's *you* who must judge the rightness or wrongness of a situation, whether it's in your household or in your government, and decide how it's to be remedied, if you believe it wrong. And it's *you* whose mind determines the nature of the surroundings in your family—use it to your fullest advantage. Be aware of what you are, where you're going, and what you're doing. Be aware of what your kids feel and do and think. You may prevent a tragedy in your household!

HOW HEALTH HABITS CAN WORK TO YOUR ADVANTAGE AND DISADVANTAGE

You have begun to form good habits if you're controlling your blood sugar levels through diet, physical conditioning and mind control. If you've sloughed any of these three important keystones of efficient blood sugar control, you're still a servant to old bad habits.

How Iris Got Control of Her Mind Through Blood Sugar Control

A middle-aged lady, I'll call her Iris, had this trouble. She had always had a problem in relating to other people—she was an intelligent woman, but sounded like a dolt whenever she had to talk to someone, be it a group of friends, her relatives, or even her family. She "clammed-up" when she had to expose any part of her "self" to others. She'd become much overweight, sluggish, and avoided physical activity of all kinds. Iris literally ate her way to satisfaction, not finding relief in her personal relationships.

She'd tried dieting using drugs and no exercise many times in the past, always ending in a complete flop. She'd tried personality courses, also ending in failure. *When she was convinced that her trouble basically was in poor habits of blood sugar control, she began to make headway.* First, she began a program of exercise and diet in the manner I've discussed in previous sections. Her health immediately improved with diminished weight and flab. Secondly, she began to gain control of her mind and realized very quickly that her trouble started as a young girl at which time she was continually "put down" by her parents and older brothers and sisters. Thirdly, she substituted good habits for bad—she began to make herself talk to others. She began to put herself into positions where she had to talk. She volunteered to address the PTA at school. She volunteered to talk to a small study group at the church to which she belonged. And she began to "bring out" members of her family—to artfully lead them into conversation. In short, Iris began to substitute good habits of mind for the bad ones she'd acquired over the years. The results were amazing. She became so good at conversation that she is now in demand to give book readings all over town. People actually seek her out to talk over problems, projects, and just to hear her opinion on community matters.

The way to correct a bad habit is to substitute a good one in its place. This is an old remedy, but it works like a charm. Try it. You'll be dieting, exercising and controlling your *blood sugar levels* in a short time. There's no limit to what you may accomplish!

YOUR MIND AND EXTRA-SENSORY PERCEPTION

One of the most fascinating areas in the study of mind is that of ESP—extra-sensory perception. This means knowing, but without the use of the five senses. Hence the term "sixth sense." The possibility of such an act—of knowing without seeing, hearing, feeling, tasting or smelling—has been challenged by the scientific community for years. Yet ESP does exist: How could it? This question has given birth to a new science: Parapsychology, the scientific study of ESP. Parapsychology is young and still suffers the bigotry of the skeptical establishment. But it's coming to the fore.

In the first place, it should be noted that the dedicated scientists in the field of parapsychology have *proven* that there exists telepathy, clairvoyance, psychokinesis and retroscopy.

TELEPATHY. The sensation of knowing the thoughts of another and of causing another to know your thoughts is called telepathy. This occurs without the spoken, written or physically transmitted signal. Do thoughts you have in your mind travel? Can some people pick them up? How are they transmitted? In waves? In as yet not understood physical "current"? The answers to these questions aren't known yet, but parapsychologists are working on them. The field is new; it's exciting. And parapsychology will likely take its proper place among the respected sciences within the next decade.

CLAIRVOYANCE. Clairvoyance is the ability to see events before they've occurred. The term, *precognition,* is more often used today to describe this peculiar ability: A "knowing beforehand" is what the word means. How would it be possible to know something before it happened? A perfectly logical question. All I can say is that the late Dr. Albert Einstein caused us to revise our usual opinions concerning cause and effect with his theories of relativity. Among others, his concepts give us reason to believe that what has happened in the past, what is happening now, and what will happen tomorrow are all somehow related in a here-and-now way; that we are "imbedded," so to speak, in an already-formed space-time fabric about which we actually know very little in spite of our super-science. Our sub-conscious mind—perhaps it might be better called our paraconscious mind—may well be attuned to this space-time flux—it may be able to sense, in other words, Einstein's space-time continuum. If this is true, it's easier to see why clairvoyance is neither mysterious nor impossible. If the space in which we exist is sensible to the mind, why not time as well? The common hunch or intuition is partly clairvoyant in nature.

PSYCHOKINESIS. The influence of mind over matter is psycho-kinesis. This issue is the hottest debated of all ESP phenomena. On the surface, influencing matter may seem like a fairy-tale. But it's not. Consider this: If you can "will" yourself either to turn the next page of this book or not as you decide, are you not influencing matter with your mind? When your fingers actually turn the page at your direction, certainly your mind has influenced matter in the form of nerve and muscle tissue. To carry it outward another step, when you influence another person, perhaps your four-year-old child, that 2 + 2 adds up to 4, are you not influencing his mind with yours? And since your child's mind is composed of matter (nerve tissue, brain cells and the like) are you not influencing matter with your mind? Try influencing the throw of ordinary dice—concentrate on a particular combination and have someone else throw for you—it may surprise you that you can, sometimes, call the throws! Practice will improve this to a certain degree. At this point, no one knows how far such influence can be carried, but it is under investigation.

RETROSCOPY. Retroscopy is a term meaning that a person has the ability to sense what has happened in the past. This is the ability to have sensations of knowing by handling a personal object belonging to a person who may now be dead or missing. It's the opposite of clairvoyance. It's a matter of common knowledge that in certain European countries, people that have the ability of retroscopy are *routinely* sought by police departments to help solve missing persons, murder cases and other cases because their results have been so universally correct in the past!

SUMMARY

1. Think of your body and mind as a single unit—the one must be present for the other to exist. You can't influence one with-out influencing the other. Now that you are getting your body into shape with proper diet and exercise routines, your mind is already growing and increasing its power.
2. The key to increasing your mind power is concentration. Con-centration develops will power. Learn to increase your will

power by learning to concentrate. In this way, you will have more mind output.

3. There is tremendous potential in your sub-conscious mind. Since one of its jobs is to store the everyday happenings in your life, you will want to learn how some of this stored material can be retrieved. Concentration, together with autosuggestion, will help you do this.

4. Proper habits of mind come as a result of substituting good habits of mind for bad ones. Autosuggestion and concentration can help you make such substitutions. When you learn this technique, you can use them to increase your efficiency in diet and physical conditioning which, in turn, will increase your mind control.

5. The science of extra-sensory perception is new and can add to your mind control since you may increase your own ESP with practice. Many hunches and intuitions are forms of ESP trying to "get through" to your conscious mind.

6

How to Maintain Sparkling Health Through Better Blood Sugar Control

How is your health? Want to improve it—tone up your body and mind so that they're working at peak performance? I'm going to show you how to do that in this chapter. I'm going to discuss with you how to make the air you breathe work better to your advantage, explain about proper rest and relaxation, and how it guards your total health.

I think the problem of drugs is also important, so they, too, will come under examination in this section.

It's time we took a look at your lungs and kidneys—how they work and how to keep them in top order. Along with these vital organs, I'm going to you show you what you can do to prevent disease in joints, tendons and muscles. We will also look at the problem of allergy and what you can do about it.

The role of your blood sugar level and its effect on stomach and intestinal disease is important to your good health. I will discuss with you ways you can keep your digestive organs in good running order.

The constant battle your body wages with invading germs and viruses relates to how well you maintain blood sugar levels. I will show you what you can do about avoiding infection. Finally, the problem of cancer—what you may do to avoid it and how to watch for it.

HOW TO BREATHE A BETTER SUPPLY OF VITAL OXYGEN

The broad relation of the cells in your body, your blood sugar and your oxygen supply has been pointed out in previous chapters. Given a cell whose metabolism is at peak and a blood sugar level that's optimal—these two vital states then need one more link for the chain of life: A constant source of oxygen. These three links combine to make the human life cycle complete. It then remains for your system to eliminate the waste products of such a "biological furnace," and the life cycle begins anew.

Your body has only one effective way to get oxygen: You breathe it in from the surrounding air. Air, of course, isn't pure oxygen— you really don't need pure oxygen, thanks to nature's ingenious method of extracting it from a mixture inside your lungs. Remember our discussion in Chapter 3 of the constant need in your body of a source of animal protein? Besides the protein in meat, you get a good supply of iron, the element that your body uses to make red blood cells. These special cells carry oxygen from your lungs to all your body cells. So there are four main points to think about with your oxygen supply.

1. The air you breathe.
2. The condition of the air pump that takes in the air.
3. The condition of the membranes inside the millions of tiny air sacs in your lungs.
4. The transport system for the oxygen: Your red blood cells.

AIR. There is much controversy today about air pollution. I'm certain that if enough foreign material gets into our air, it causes ill-health. Cities like New York, Pittsburgh and Los Angeles have had the problem for a number of years, but there is as yet no conclusive evidence that all the people who live in large cities suffer over the long haul. No doubt exists that on some days many people *do* suffer temporarily. But the long range effects on general health are difficult to demonstrate. Someday, they may very well be proven. Meanwhile, air pollution remains an irritating, distressing, sometimes noxious thorn in the side of our civilized cities. The air you breathe in, however, still has about the same concentration of vital oxygen it always has had. This in spite of drastically increased use from the swelling world population.

I think more damage is done the citizenry of this country by what they do in their homes and offices concerning air than occurs in all outdoors. Most people don't realize their homes and offices need a *constant* supply of *fresh* air in order for them to maintain adequate levels of blood sugar and oxygen. Fresh air demands new air brought *in* from outside and stale air returned *to* the outside. Figures show more people suffocate from a lack of this free interchange of air than from the effects of pollution. Every winter, in every city, entire families are overcome by fumes from improperly ventilated furnaces, stoves and heaters. If there had been adequate exchange of air from the outside, such accidents would have been and could be prevented. The faulty vent involved, of course, needs to be corrected, *but so does the air exchange inside your house.* The simple way to do this is always to have one or more windows open, even in subzero temperature, somewhere in your house—especially at night!

YOUR AIR PUMP. There is a large muscle in your body that separates your chest cavity from your abdominal cavity called the diaphragm. Your diaphragm is the main muscle of breathing—it's nothing more than a large bellows that sucks in and blows out air. Learning to use your diaphragm efficiently helps deliver a better supply of air to your lungs.

To people who use their voices for a living—like singers and lecturers—the diaphragm breathes for them through their abdomens primarily. Take a normal breath and watch your chest and abdomen. Does only your chest expand with this inspiration? If so, you're using your diaphragm inefficiently. This time, take in your breath by making your abdomen pooch out first, then expand your chest. Note how much more air gets in this way. Note also how much more waste air (carbon dioxide) is pushed out. This is proper breathing. Practice this method before a mirror or until you get the feel of abdominal breathing. You'll keep more alert, have better blood sugar levels, and will be more healthy for the effort.

Your exercise routine, already started by now, will automatically tone your diaphragm as you breath rapidly from the exertion, whether it be from walking, calisthenics, isometrics or weight lifting. So don't worry about the tone of your diaphragm, it's well cared for by any exercise routine. But learn to breathe with your abdomen and by chest expansion during exercises. You'll be amazed how this will pay off with increased stamina and endurance.

YOUR AIR SAC MEMBRANES. In your lungs, the arteries and veins branch hundreds of times like the branches of a tree until they reach such small size that only a single chain of red blood cells can travel down their tube-like interiors. These tiny microscopic vessels are called capillaries. Capillaries wrap themselves around the tiny grape-like air sacs, and it's here, across a membrane so thin that it's all but invisible, where oxygen passes into your bloodstream and carbon dioxide (the waste from cell metabolism) passes out. Since both oxygen and carbon dioxide are in a gaseous state, the transfer is rapid and quite efficient. Rapid and efficient, that is, unless this thin wispy membrane is diseased and has thickened for any number of reasons.

You have already undertaken the first method in keeping these important membranes in good repair with your exercise routines. The forced breathing started by increasing your muscular endurance is expanding and contracting all those small muscles that control the air sac size and tone. The second method for healthy air sacs is the gathering in of plenty of fresh outside air—by breathing with your abdomen and enjoying physical activity out of doors. The third rule is that of forcing in eight to ten deep breaths at least four times during the day—stop whatever it is you may be doing to breathe as deeply as you can. You will completely change all the air in the tiny sacs. Normal breathing doesn't quite exchange the air in the sacs, but *forced deep* breathing *will* exchange this stale air and increase the efficiency of oxygen transport.

The last rule to remember concerning air sac membranes is that excessive smoking *definitely damages their membranes*. Your smoking should be cut 50 per cent today, and if possible, another 25 per cent over the following two or three weeks. You have learned at least three ways to help you with this: Will power, autosuggestion, and the substitution of one habit for another.

When you have the urge to smoke, do the abdominal breathing exercises instead. You can drift off to sleep at night concentrating on the suggestion that you won't crave smoking and that you will smoke less as time passes. You may substitute drinking a glass of skim milk or having a snack instead of that next cigarette.

YOUR RED BLOOD CELLS. Most routine physical examinations today call for the simple measure of the number of red blood cells in your body by the measurement of iron or a similar test. If you have a shortage of iron—in other words, are anemic—your doctor will reverse this state of affairs by appropriate measures. You can insure a continuing supply of iron by taking in enough protein in your diet. This is automatically accomplished, remember, by having ample meat in your diet.

SECRETS OF RELAXATION REVEALED

Over the years, I've waged a running battle with people who don't take time to relax, and with institutions who can't see that their employees would work with about 50 per cent more efficiency if they had more time away from work.

How a Housewife Benefited from Effective Relaxation

A lady I'll call Edna is typical of women who must number in the tens of thousands of housewives in this country. Edna, because she hadn't learned how to control blood sugar, came into the office repeatedly, each time with a new complaint or a new symptom. She was already taking three different pills for the most recent of her aches and pains. Actually, there wasn't anything physically wrong with Edna except that she was bored. Her children were in school and she found herself with too much idle time. The television soap operas and magazine love stories soon failed to hold her attention. She began to focus most of her attention onto herself. She hadn't the least idea how to relax and rest properly, or how to put her mind to work productively.

The first thing I did was ask her to stop taking all the pills. Next, I taught Edna how to exercise and diet—she was about 30 pounds overweight, and her chest and abdominal muscles suffered the neglect so common in women after childbirth. When Edna began to melt away her aches and other symptoms, we had a long talk. Edna was bright and alert, but she'd never extended herself beyond her immediate household and family. The clubs and activities she'd wrapped herself up in weren't really what she wanted to be doing. Edna told me during one of our talks that she'd always wanted to do something creative like writing or painting, but she figured it was futile to try either one. Furthermore, she believed her family might laugh her out of the house if she tried. What nonsense! I encouraged her to join a local writer's club I happened to know. Edna found, much to her surprise, that there were a whole raft of people, some nearby in her own neighborhood, who had the same interest. She began to learn something about the field of writing and began to do something she really wanted to do. She soon forgot her aches and pains and is today a healthy vigorous person, and she takes no drugs whatever.

Relaxation means different things to different people. To some, comfortable relaxation would seem sheer drudgery to others, and hard work to still others. The point is, when you get ready to rest and relax, do the things that interest *you*. Not useless gyrations you might think others would like to see you doing. If this means joining a sun-bathing colony or becoming a hair stylist, do it. Just spend your spare time *doing* it, and throw yourself into it heart and soul.

The Beating Breadwinners Take

The man, or woman, who supports the family and brings home the bacon is subject to all kinds of pressures and stress. This is life—stress is beautifully compatible with a long and healthy life at that, in spite of what you may have heard. Pressure is what makes the world go around. And it's what increases the amount of bacon available for bringing home! But everyone has his limits. No one can stay hard at this business of work without frequent breaks, and remain either productive or healthy.

Consider Charley, who works at a production line in a factory. In spite of the fact that his union has provided good benefits, including vacation time, for him and his fellow-workers, Charley puts off vacations until a specific time, usually in late summer. This he does for a variety of reasons. He has children in school, and they can't be yanked out any old time to go somewhere. Then when summer starts, the kids wrap themselves up in programs that require their presence for so many weeks, and on it goes. Besides, Charley hasn't the money to spend on two or three jaunts a year. When vacation times does come around, it's a marathon. A test of stamina and endurance to see whether Charley and his wife and three kids can drive 5000 miles and visit all the relatives and see all the sights in two weeks. When I talked to such a Charley not long ago, he was bored, he was irritable and listless, and his ambition had flagged some time in the past and hadn't returned.

Eventually, Charley found he didn't have to travel to Tahiti or make a Canadian safari to enjoy his earned vacation time. He finally learned that there was more to spending an evening than sitting in front of the television set, or going to a movie, or just napping after dinner. Charley always thought he could become interested in photography, but he'd never given it a whirl. Once started, he found he was pretty good at it. Charley's wife was quite a seamstress. Between them, they devised a way to imprint her original patterns photographically so they could be duplicated easily. So popular was their newly found hobby that Charley and his wife are seriously considering going into business for themselves—if for no other reason than that they are both doing something they are intensely interested in and enjoy, and they'll undoubtedly make a go of it.

THE NECESSITY FOR REST

And there's a time to rest. I mean, really rest. On the flat of your back with your eyes shut. Your muscles and your brain tell you when this time is at hand. Sleep is something that depends on individual make-up—the unique body-mind combination that's yours alone. I've known people who have trained themselves to go to sleep almost within seconds, given concentration and practice. Some of these people report that if they go to sleep for about two minutes in the middle of the day, their energy and stamina are increased threefold for the day. You have probably met people who seem to need only four or five hours of sleep a night, while you may require ten to twelve hours for full efficiency. This is part of that uniqueness again, but with practice, you can cut the amount of sleep you need if you use your mind's automatic alarm to wake up earlier.

Psychologists tell us that during sleep, the human mind goes through a kind of "unwinding process." That the mind takes advantage of sleep to reshuffle and reorganize things according to what occurred during the preceding waking hours. Dreams seem to be a part of this reshuffling. So dream away and don't worry about dreaming or about your kids who talk a lot during sleep—it's better not to interrupt talking or dreaming sleepers.

If you just can't find the time during the day, two good times for relaxing are just after lunch and supper. Seek out a couch or lounge, put your feet up on a stool or table, and let every muscle in your body go completely limp. Close your eyes and with your newly developed concentration ability, put everything out of your mind, even if it's only for five minutes. You'll notice the change immediately, in the form of increased energy, alertness and productivity.

DRUGS: THE GREAT AMERICAN INSTITUTION

I wonder about responsible parents who in one breath cry out in mortal agony at the "alarming rate of drug abuse" among youngsters today, and in the very next are, themselves, taking from four to six pills, pouring down a pitcher full of martinis at noon and again in the evening, and who are smoking their lungs out of existence. What might we expect? Parents, fortunately or unfortunately, are no longer in a position to tell their children one thing, but do another themselves. The day of the double standard of conduct is no longer going to be tolerated by youngsters, and I believe it's about time.

But the drug abuse goes on—aided and abetted by our present age of miracle drugs and by people who are in too much of a hurry to put up with anything but instant cure of all ills with drugs. We've become a pill-happy group of people in this country.

We physicians have done little to counteract this trend, but I'm afraid the day is here when we must deal with the problem.

I'm not advocating that we discard the corner or supermarket drug store. Far from this, I'm simply advocating *restraint* with your drug-taking habits. There are many drugs that are constantly overused in medical practice. I'd like to discuss a few of the more common offenders.

THYROID. Thyroid extract, and all of the more recently discovered synthetic thyroid compounds, are flagrantly overused and misused by the pill-conscious American today. The overweight housewife and working girl are the most outstanding examples of this drug fraud. The last poor woman I saw with the problem was taking six grains of thyroid extract every day. Enough for a dozen patients with valid reason for taking thyroid! This woman was overweight all right, but had been told, "Your thyroid gland is probably underactive." No tests were given to find out. When I first saw the lady, she was so nervous from the side effect of thyroid extract intoxication that she was nearly incapacitated and her husband had contacted a psychiatrist for therapy! Fortunately, her nervousness subsided after stopping the drug, and her weight problem was handled effectively by methods I've already discussed.

Don't take thyroid unless tests *prove its need!* It will do *nothing* about your weight, and may, in fact, cause so much tension and anxiety that your weight may go up.

HEART STIMULANTS. These very potent drugs are now "in" for weight reduction and a host of other run-down conditions, as well as for tonics to "pep you up." Some idiots have actually combined them with thyroid for "added stimulation and prompt effect"! Digitalis preparations are the commonly used drugs with such tonic. This combination can only be regarded as poison! Digitalis is a dangerous drug, and it takes experienced physicians years to completely master its use. Does it make any sense at all to gorge on such a drug without expert guidance? Emphatically *no!* The last patient I knew who had taken such a preparation for weight loss was a middle-aged man whose heart sustained such damage that he spent a month in the hospital recuperating from cardiac standstill—in other words, this famous tonic had caused his heart to stop beating for a short time. He recovered, no thanks to his medicine.

Quinidine, another heart drug, in some ways more potent and in every way more toxic than digitalis, is currently in vogue for treating people with every imaginable ailment, including of all things, spastic colon! Today there aren't more than three indications for this drug, and these are for tricky heart conditions for which heart specialists insist their patients be hospitalized before starting treatment. Don't take any digitalis or quinidine-containing medicine except under an expert's watchful eye!

TRANQUILIZERS. As might have been predicted, its's now become fashionable to take a pill to solve problems that we have actually created. I'm talking about the so-called stresses and strains of daily living. We have pills to pep up, pills to calm down, pills to normalize, pills to sedate, pills to sleep, pills to—who knows what next? The trouble I find with this class of medicines is that it's a little like treating the skin rash that appears with typhoid fever—you may have a beautiful skin cure, but the patient may succumb from the disease which, of course, is untouched by the efforts on his skin. We aren't getting to sources with the drugs. We are curing the nerves, but leaving the patient to rot with his mental strife, whatever it may be.

And don't be misled by statistics from mental hospitals. Sure, they've been able to cut their hospital beds over the past ten years, *but there are more people seen at mental hospitals than ever*. They're just keeping more and more of them on a modified out-patient status than was possible before the age of tranquilizers. In general, take tranquilizers with caution, under expert supervision and on a limited time basis, unless you've been *admitted* to a mental hospital.

The Case of a Middle-Aged Heart Patient

Many of our drug problems are strictly a matter of the way medical care is given in certain areas. Unfortunately, it's the financially not-so-well-off patient who most often gets into this mess.

Consider a patient I saw at a neighborhood health center project set up under the poverty program in a large metropolitan city not long ago. Bill, I'll call him, was typical of thousands in his spot. He was middle-aged and usually went to the city general hospital for his ills. Here, he saw a different doctor each time, when he managed to be seen, that is. Bill had a heart condition. The ailment needed two drugs taken in low doses over long periods of time to hold it in check and keep Bill feeling well. Over the past three years, Bill had collected no less than 15 different drugs, some for the same symptoms, others for symptoms that Bill could have gotten relief from with much simpler, short-term therapy. But every time he'd mention a new sign or symptom to the general hospital doctors, he'd get more pills.

When I saw him, he was confused, sick and overdrugged. None of the many doctors who had seen Bill in the hospital clinics had access to Bill's previous records, or else they didn't have time to look at them. If they had, this sorry situation wouldn't have occurred. This case points up a very hypocritical situation long overdue for correction: These same doctors getting their training by practicing on tens of thousands of Bills in the country would no more tolerate such practice in their middle-class patients than they would fly. Why, then, does this horribly sloppy state of affairs continue in every city general hospital in the country? The answer is based on poor judgment of the needs of people when they're sick—there just "isn't time" to spare the sick indigent, but always plenty of time when a paying patient is calling the shots!

This problem isn't limited to city general hospitals; I've seen it happen in private practice. Again, doctors won't take the time to find out what drugs their patients have been taking, and patients won't take the time to tell doctors what's in the bathroom medicine chest at home.

The time is with us that we need fewer drugs and more treatment. *You need to depend less on medicines and more on keeping your blood sugar up to par.* If you do, you'll find far less need for pills. If you have to take more than four different drugs, regardless of the complexity of your conditions, you should see if you can start reducing the number. If you have peculiar reactions that you can definitely date to about the time you started taking any drugs, bring it to the attention of your doctor—find out if the drug is really necessary. *Drugs may stand between you and efficient control of your blood sugar!*

HOW TO KEEP YOUR INTERNAL ORGANS IN GOOD ORDER

Kidneys

The parts of your body that eliminate waste are important to maintaining blood sugar levels. Your kidneys are the major part of your body's filter system. As blood flows through your kidneys, the greater part of the liquid portion of your blood is removed entirely, run through the filters, the chemicals needed by your body returned, and the waste materials excreted in your urine. Working in this way, your kidneys have almost absolute control over the salt and water balance, the concentration of all the minerals in your blood, the conservation of necessary proteins and other nutriments and the amounts of toxic wastes in your body at any given time. Remember the following in keeping your kidneys efficient in their work:

A Program for Kidney Care

1. Drink plenty of all kinds of liquids all day, every day of the week and every week of the month. Your kidneys depend on water to do their job. This is especially important in hot weather and during hard physical work such as your exercise routines because of water lost through perspiration.
2. You can't strain your kidneys if they're working properly. They're built to do the special job they perform. Better to be going to the bathroom more frequently than to spare them of doing their job.
3. If you have any reason to believe your urinary tract isn't functioning right, see a medical expert. The smell of urine doesn't mean a thing. Go by how you feel. If there is pain or an urgency to go to the bathroom even though no urine or only a tiny bit is forthcoming, this is vastly more significant than urine odor.

4. Women, particularly those with large families, are prone to have mechanical difficulties with their urinary apparatus. This can be corrected. If you seem to be leaking urine when you cough or exert, or if you can't control your bladder too well, this is the most likely trouble. Your kidneys are all right, though, and a simple repair can correct the condition.

5. In men, prostate trouble often first manifests itself in difficulty with urinating or with bladder control. If such symptoms occur, don't delay being examined by an expert.

The point to remember in these *lower* urinary troubles is that, if neglected, they can begin to damage your kidneys. It isn't wise to postpone treatment.

Care of Lungs

I've discussed the role of the lungs in connection with oxygen intake. They are vulnerable to abuse because every time you take in a breath, the air sucked in has to contact their linings. Whenever something is burning or smoking, the fumes can be assumed to be irritating your lungs. Many factories and all mining industries have this problem among their workers. The cities everywhere are faced with the problem in the form of smog. If you live in an area where smog is a problem, you work in a factory with fume problems, and you smoke, you can almost take odds that your lungs will eventually suffer. It's amazing, actually, what your lungs will take without acting up. Give them a break. Cut back severely on your cigarette smoking. Switch to a pipe. Get adequate ventilation at home and at work.

The numbers of people in this country with a disease called emphysema show a steady increase each year. Emphysema starts when those little air sacs are no longer able to contract during the breathing out part of your respiration cycle. They dilate like a balloon and cause poor oxygen exchange. A patient with this disease will start to notice trouble any time after he is forty years old or so. At first, a little shortness of breath with exertion may be all you notice. Gradually, this increases until ordinary walking causes you to huff and puff like a steam engine. Repeated bouts of bronchitis and the changes this brings add themselves to the picture. Soon, emphysema makes a lung cripple of you—unable to breathe properly at all, an invalid, and a mighty unhappy person in general. Don't let yourself slip into this picture. Keep your "internal pollution" at the lowest possible degree by paying attention to what your doctor tells you about your smoking, your working conditions, and even your place of residence. And exercise! Keep those air sacs in good condition.

Joints and Muscles

If you put a perfectly well arm or leg in a plaster cast for six weeks, all the joints that are immobilized will be stiff, and the muscles that move them sore, weak and shrunken. Anyone who has had a broken bone will remember this picture very well. The point is, to maintain their functional abilities, joints and muscles *must be used*. An injury may require splinting or casting. But when the injury is healed, the first thing, and the hardest, that must be overcome is stiff joints and shrunken muscles. You can help prevent arthritis by what you've already started—your physical conditioning routines. Exercise not only keeps your joints limber, but also strengthens the muscles and ligaments so that injury and strain are far less likely, reducing even further the chances of arthritis.

Notice an older person with stiff weak joints. What has he done? He's been too inactive! If he'd been active, had good nutrition, and trained his mind to keep him perking, his joints wouldn't be nearly so stiff. Not all arthritis can be prevented, but much of it can. Keep limber; keep moving.

Deforming arthritis, the kind that makes fingers, legs and backs twisted and useless, is partly hereditary and partly caused from stress. If it develops, all isn't lost. You can learn to get along quite nicely with the uninvolved joints and muscles. And if there's ever a place for having prepared yourself with good blood sugar control, it's at the time when this type of arthritis (rheumatoid arthritis) appears. If your weight, muscle tone and mind have been attuned and are functioning at optimal level, your chances of fighting rheumatoid arthritis are increased a hundred times. If there has been neglect in any of these areas of body and mind, the disease can become quite troublesome. Another of hundreds of reasons to start whipping your blood sugar into shape *now!*

Minimizing Allergies

The allergic state is caused by the fact that your system is sensitive to a variety of things that are eaten, breathed in, or that get into you by way of bacteria. The common allergy is the variety that touches off your nose, eyes, and throat when particular dusts, pollens and other inhalants are breathed in. This is the variety known as hay-fever. Why the cells in your nose or eyes and no others would react to such breathed-in substances has been a curious mystery in past years. It's now known that the breathed-in substances cause a reaction like that produced by your body in response to an infection. And it's the antibodies your body produces against the invader material that raise cain with your nose and eyes.

How to Cope with Hay Fever

If you start getting control of your blood sugar, you've already started the way to improved times with allergies, if you happen to suffer them. *It's surprising what you can do with blood sugar control in handling allergies.* If you're a hay-fever sufferer, for example, your trouble is mostly watery red and irritated eyes, itching running noses and sneezing. You can do as a young woman I know who went through this agony from spring to the first frost of fall (when offending weeds are finally killed). Understanding that the symptoms in her head were primarily produced by dilated blood vessels—causing the running nose and watery eyes—she was able to control her symptoms very much as did the patient with migraine discussed previously (note the similarity in the problem of dilated blood vessels). When she felt a seizure coming on, she concentrated on the blood vessels in her nose and eyes. She made them constrict. And it worked! She also found she could prevent sneezing by concentrating in the same manner on the vessels in her breathing tree.

This lady didn't cure her allergies by such control, but she reduced her symptoms by 75 per cent. At first she found that her symptom control lasted only a short while—a half hour or so. As she continued to mobilize her mind behind the problem, and as she began to use autosuggestion at night, her control could be made, she learned, to last six to eight hours, as long as the antihistamine medicine she'd used!

How to Cope with Hives

I'm also acquainted with a man who was afflicted with hives whenever he ate any one of several foods. He was also allergic to penicillin and two other antibiotics. When he learned how to control his blood sugar, and when his mind was brought to bear on the problem, he found he could make the hives disappear. He understood that a hive, an itching red welt on the skin often popping out at points where clothing exerts pressure, such as the waistline or the feet, is caused by the sudden dilation—expansion—of blood vessels in a localized area of skin. As did the previous two patients, he concentrated on these blood vessels and caused them to constrict. The hives would promptly disappear. He hadn't cured the allergy responsible for the hives, but he'd learned to rid himself of the main symptom of them. He ultimately learned to do without the offending foods through diet control. You can learn these and other controls just as did these people. Faithfully following a diet, exercise, and mind control are what you need.

Care of Stomach and Intestines

The human gut is concerned with the digestion, assimilation and elimination processes. As such, its smooth function is essential to your blood sugar maintenance. If there is one place in your body where nervous energy is constantly and forcefully directed, it's your intestinal tract. Remember Chapter 3 where I discussed with you the problem of appetite? And in Chapter 4, the discussion of how your mind can bury some uncomfortable experience? Well, it's through your stomach and intestine that these two forces, appetite and buried nervous energy, are finally sidetracked—your mind discharges its tensions, anxieties and excess energy through the large nerves that control the activity of your intestinal tract! It's no wonder that stomach ulcers and spastic colons are so common! It's almost as though nature had provided for the elimination of "waste products of mind" as well as for food.

Ninety per cent of all the grief one hears about with reference to the stomach and bowels are preventable with good habits of blood sugar control. Take acid indigestion, the most common affliction of the human stomach. Your stomach always warns you of this vexing condition—you get heartburn. This is to say, you have a feeling that you just swallowed a plateful of chili peppers whole, and they're burning the lining of your stomach. The burning is a true description of what's happening—the acid that's normally in your stomach to digest food finds nothing to work on, so it works on the stomach lining. The natural end-point of continuous and repeated heartburn is a stomach ulcer.

If some foods you regularly have in your diet give you heartburn, throw them out! There may be several different things that burn, but most people know three or four foods that consistently give them indigestion. Eat, as we've previously discussed, as though you were always trying to give your stomach a break—have mid-morning and afternoon snacks. Eat in a *relaxed* atmosphere always, and don't bolt your food down as though it were your last meal. If heartburn occurs—usually following meals—do something to stop it. Use antacids freely and regularly if necessary. There are many antacids available at the drugstore not requiring a prescription, and their only action is inside your stomach. Milk of magnesia is excellent. Baking soda is a *poor* antacid. You may have days you have to use antacids six times a day—if so, use it! You'll find skimmed milk an excellent buffer—often it's as much as you need for mild heartburn. Use milk with antacids when necessary.

Spastic Colon

The spastic colon, often called an irritable gut, usually comes on some hours after eating, and is a product of poor dietary habits and a nervous disposition. Search for offending foods in this condition by eliminating from your diet first one type of food then another for two to three weeks at a time. Then bring what you know about *blood sugar control* into play—basic diet principles are a must, especially the smaller main meals and the snacks. Physical exercise is also *a must*. Your exercise routine brings about a discharge of that nervous energy over the nerves to your muscles rather than through those to your stomach. Mind control is essential because you can now begin to concentrate on the muscles that surround your intestines and cause them to *relax* with practice.

I've seen recently three patients with upper and lower intestinal problems of long standing who brought their miserable conditions under excellent control utilizing nothing more than the elements of *blood sugar control* we've discussed. One of these patients, a middle-aged woman, had been plagued by cramps and diarrhea for years, had been thoroughly examined and tested, and was used to taking six pills a day to stop her discomfort. She learned to control both the diarrhea and cramps in the space of three months. She had to lose weight, tone up flabby muscles, and learn mind control to do it. You've already begun to use these tools—put them to use in controlling your intestinal tract!

The other two patients, both young men, had already developed ulcers, and one had part of his stomach surgically removed because of complications from his ulcer. Both these men had atrocious eating habits—meals were orgies and alcohol was drunk like water—every meal was a gluttonous debauch in which not only did they gorge food, but gorged with the most rich and indigestible type of foods imaginable. Fried, greasy and fatty food were taken with gusto. Spices and condiments (catsup, mustard, relish and the like) were used by the plateful. Both were heavy smokers. And these men were used to burying a lot of nervous energy every day at their jobs and with their families—all of it went right down to their stomachs already overloaded from terrible diet habits! Neither patient has been bothered with abdominal complaints for two years. And they won't be unless they forget what they learned about blood sugar control!

Care of Infections

People in the medical profession are just beginning to learn about the human body's defenses against infection. We understand much better, and always have, how to treat infections than we do about their production in the first place. For example, it has just recently been learned that cases of pneumonia are invariably preceded by virus invasion. Remember the case of the patient I discussed previously who virtually eliminated his three or four a year chest infection problem by reducing smoking and taking up blood sugar control as part of his everyday routine? What happened was he stopped having virus infections in his chest—and the lowered resistance that brought on the bacterial infections.

And the case I discussed of the lady who was the "runt" in her family? Remember how she began to show vastly improved resistance to infections when she began muscle toning? You can practically eliminate infection from invading your system by simply following the rules of blood sugar control. Have you ever seen a well-conditioned athlete with infection problems? I haven't. The rare ones that do occur can be traced, and the athletes will be the first to admit it, to a departure from their physical fitness routines!

No doubt about it, good muscle toning *does* improve your defense mechanisms against infection. Doing sit-ups, for example, is known to empty the liver of its blood and get it into the circulation at a tremendously increased rate. The liver has cells in it that are concerned with the manufacture of those antibodies we've discussed. The ones, remember, that "read" the presence of bacteria and viruses in your body and block them from causing trouble. There are probably other factors as well that we have not as yet discovered that are brought to bear against infection when muscles are kept in good tone. The point is that *it works*. It will work for you as you gain control of your blood sugar levels.

Cancer

There are a number of things about this dread disease that aren't stressed nearly enough, though science today strives mightily to find the cure for it. The basic defect in cancer is that the particular cells involved, among all those trillions in your organism, have *lost their ability to restrain growth*. Consider for a moment the growing child—or even the developing fetus from the first day that a male sperm unites with a female egg. Consider the growth involved from the original one cell to the trillions of which your body is composed. What fantastic unimaginable growth! But when the human body reaches its proper size, this growth *must stop*. If it didn't, and we continued to grow at the same rate after our birth as we did before it, we would be nine or ten feet tall by the time we were one year old! With cancer, it appears that whatever the factors that put the brakes on cell growth as we reach adulthood are suddenly reactivated. This propensity to divide and grow into existence again in a localized area of cells results in cancer.

Take lung cancer, for example. There is no doubt today that this particular cancer—more common in men than women, and more common in city than in country dwellers—bears a definite relation to what we inhale into our chest. Everything known about lung cancer points to this relation: More common in heavy smokers than in non-smokers; more common in men (who smoke more and who work in polluted air more) than in women; more common in heavy industralized countries than in rural-based societies; and more common in age groups above 45. There is something that has to do with aging and environment in lung cancer, as well as with other cancers. It is concerned with cells that are stressed a lot in the ordinary course of events (the lungs are vulnerable to everything in the air we breathe, and the female breast is constantly stimulated by hormonal variation every week of the month). Add yet another stress factor—and one has cancer. The point is that it is the extra stress factors that can be brought under control by blood sugar surveillance.

You can control or eliminate certain disadvantageous environmental conditions that subject some of your body cells to undue pressure. If your family tree, for example, contains males that have had lung cancer, you *can* put a stop to the internal pollution of your own lungs by avoiding working conditions that make you inhale toxic or irritating fumes. You *can* refrain completely from smoking cigarettes. You *can* keep your body and mind in optimum condition by adhering to the blood sugar control methods outlined in this book. And you *can* make it part of your regular check-up twice a year to have your chest X-rayed after you reach the age of 40.

What to Do About Aspects of Cancer

The point to remember is that the foregoing discussion can apply to any cancer. I'm not advocating that you set about to eliminate all from your environment completely. The stress from hard work, creating and exercise are not stresses that seem to trigger serious disease such as cancer. In fact, if you question very elderly people who are alert, wiry and active at the age of 85, you invariably find constant and hard application of body and mind in their backgrounds. I'm talking about the irritants that constantly inflame, infect, or otherwise break down the cells so that they must wage a battle to remain in a normal state.

Cancer of the skin is a good example of this. You can spend years working in the sunlight, wind and weather extremes, having irritated splotches appear and heal, reappear and reheal in continuous fashion. Then one day one of the splotches doesn't heal, but remains an ulcerated spot that turns into skin cancer. These splotches that have been appearing and healing—you *can* stop them. Simply by protecting your skin with emollients and sun shades (sun-tan oils and lotions), you can prevent that particular cancer! This is a prime example also of what I mean when I speak of mind and body as one—the alert mind recognizes the constant reappearance on the skin of lesions that irritate and inflame, and is stimulated into action that stops it!

SUMMARY

1. Blood sugar control and adequate oxygen supply are essential to vigorous positive metabolism. To insure yourself of a constant supply of oxygen, you must learn to breathe properly, have a continuous source of freshly circulated air to breathe, and must maintain an adequate oxygen transport system in the form of plenty of red blood cells.
2. Good health depends on adequate rest and relaxation, an activity that calls on your mastery of diet, exercise, and mind controls.
3. Drugs can do more to dampen your good health than to im-

prove it, and should be supervised by an expert or not used at all.

4. Your lungs play a vital role in every facet of blood control. The care and treatment of your lungs will produce dividends in your later years, and involves careful attention to what you breathe into them.

5. An adequate fluid balance and freedom from infection are keys to keeping your organs of elimination of wastes, your kidneys and intestines, in efficient working order. Your muscles, bones and joints will remain in good working order if you are following the tenets of *blood sugar control:* adequate diet and proper physical conditioning.

6. Allergies and infections represent immune (resistance) deficiencies. Your body can fight off such disease states if you give it a reasonable chance. Keep your blood sugar at optimum levels for this chance.

7. Control of your environment does affect the production of cancer. Your mind is now being attuned so that it recognizes the improper stresses in your surroundings. Then it's up to you to correct them to your advantage.

7

How to Spare Your Heart and Blood Vessels Needless Wear and Tear Through Blood Sugar Control

Because diseases of the heart and blood vessels cause more death and disability in America than any other disease, I want to discuss them in this chapter. You should understand what makes the heart "tick" and how to keep it working properly. Once again, the relationship between blood sugar levels and heart and blood vessel disease will be examined and how you can avoid difficulties with both. Specific heart diseases will be covered—their diagnosis and treatment. And most important, their prevention through blood sugar maintenance.

Your blood vessels are vulnerable to many influences inside and outside of your body. It's important that you know what these forces are, what to do when you recognize one or more of them, and how they're dealt with.

You live in an environment that can be controlled in regard to heart and blood vessel diseases. I will show you how some of this can be done.

Finally, there are some new techniques used to overcome heart and blood vessel disease. You should know what they are, so I'll discuss some of them in detail.

THE MOST EFFICIENT AUTOMATIC PUMP IN THE WORLD

I'd defy any engineer to come up with a manmade pump capable of continuous uninterrupted activity, without pause for repair or breakdown, and with a 5,000 plus gallon a day pumping capacity that he'd guarantee to run continuously under such circumstances for at least 70 years. Such are the impressive specifications for your heart! This magnificent piece of biological machinery deserves your special attention. Let's look closely at how your heart is put together, and what makes it work.

CONSTRUCTION OF HEART

Your heart is a muscular bag with four hollow chambers inside it. The two upper chambers are called auricles and the two lower chambers are the ventricles. The left ventricle is the largest and the strongest chamber as far as muscle strength is concerned. It's from this left ventricle that blood is pumped throughout your body. The right ventricle is quite strong, but less so than the left. It's from the right ventricle that blood is pumped into your lungs, a relatively short trip, to pick up vital oxygen. The left auricle, the upper chamber on the left side, receives this newly oxygenated blood from your lungs and empties it into the left ventricle for distribution to your body. The right auricle, the chamber on the right side above the ventricle, receives the blood from your body and empties it into the right ventricle for its journey to the lungs. Both ventricles beat at the same time, and both auricles beat at the same time. When the ventricles beat, the valves between them and the upper chambers, the auricles, are closed. The valves to the lung and body vessels are, of course, open. When the auricles beat, delivering their blood to the ventricles, the valves to the lung and body vessels are closed, and the valves between auricles and ventricles are, of course, open.

The heart, then, is a muscular bag with the bottom part built of thicker and stronger muscles than the top. It has four chambers, two inlets and two outlets, the openings to each of which are controlled by a valve.

HEART CONTROLS

The controls to this muscular blood pump are virtually auto-matic, though to a small degree capable of willed influence. There are two sets of nerves and a special set of blood vessels running through the heart. One set of nerves speeds up its rate of pumping, the other slows it down. The blood vessels to the heart are just above the opening to the outlet of the left ventricle—just beyond the valve that covers this opening when the ventricle is filling. Thus Nature insures that it is the vital heart muscle that first receives the freshly oxygenated blood as it is pumped out. In ad-dition, there are some openings in the chambers on the right side through which blood may get into the heart muscle even though blood on the right side isn't saturated yet with oxygen. This is a safeguard to insure that blood has free access to the heart under the most adverse circumstances.

Inside the heart there is a special switchboard of nerves capable of further controlling the messages it gets from the brain through the two main nerve channels.

Control of the heart, then, is through two main sets of nerves, modified by a special circuit inside the heart, and by blood vessels that reach heart muscles through both the inside and the outside of the heart wall.

A Case of "Nerves" Causing "Heart Attack"

That the nerve control to the heart can and does cause all sorts of needless concern in the form of supposed "heart attacks" was evident in a young woman I saw during a routine physical exam-ination. Rose, I'll call her, told me that she had had "six heart attacks over the past two years." I must have looked rather sur-prised at this statement. She then followed with, "Oh yes, I was in the hospital about three days with each one!" When I asked her to describe how one of her "attacks" presented itself, she told me that they invariably started during a period of nervous stress and emotion. She described how, feeling very tired, she noticed her heart suddenly doing "flip-flops," and that her pulse was fast and pounded in her head. This was followed by pain in her chest and neck. She reported also that her doctor could "tell by her EKG" (the machine used to diagnose heart disturbances) that she was actually having an "attack."

When I reviewed her EKG's, they told me what I suspected. Rose wasn't really having true heart attacks at all, but was having a trick played on her by the nerves that control her heart beat. She was having short episodes of rapid pulse brought on by nervous exhaustion, and her heart wasn't diseased or damaged in any way!

The set of nerves that speed up the heart beat were being used by her mind to carry off excess nervous energy, much like the patient discussed previously whose stomach nerves were used to do the same thing.

Such episodes of "palpitations," flip-flops, pounding, and the like are *not* heart attacks at all, but merely nervous episodes. Rose misunderstood the explanation she received about her trouble, and was living the life of a semi-invalid because she thought it best for her "bad heart." When she was convinced that all was really well with her heart, Rose brought herself out into the world and began to enjoy physical activity again. She even learned how to nip her palpitations as soon as they appeared. There is a simple reflex nerve action on the heart that can slow the beat if it's fast. You need only lie down and exert pressure with your thumbs on your closed eye balls. This maneuver is safe and can avoid much discomfort in people who go through such nervous gyrations with their hearts.

THE CONTINUOUS THREAT OF OVERWEIGHT

You're probably weary of reading about the ill-effects of being too heavy. But the point can't be emphasized enough that excess weight is the most dangerous threat to health in the country today.

As far as your heart is concerned, it is built to pump blood through the channels contained in your body in its normal amount of bone, muscle, and fatty tissues. People with heavy frames, in other words, have bigger hearts than people with light frames. Add ten, twenty or thirty pounds to these tissues and your heart must work harder, usually under conditions of decreased heart muscle tone since weight gathering isn't usual with people who are physically active. Most hearts can take this only so long—then something has to give. If your heart has reached its maximum reserve for such added weight load, it begins to give out often with disastrous results.

In addition, a certain amount of excess flab always accumulates around the heart itself—nature seems to deposit fat tissue around areas containing active muscles. Wherever fat accumulates, a new blood supply must be developed to keep it living. Around the heart, excess fat siphons off blood channels that would be better contained in the heart muscle. Remember that a heart needs all the extra blood supply it can muster if a true heart attack occurs.

More subtle, however, is the effect on general metabolism with fat accumulation. The fat person has more *circulating* fats in his blood stream than usual. It is these circulating fats, remember, that deposit themselves on the inside lining of blood vessels, including the coronary blood vessels that supply the heart muscle with its blood. Remember that when these deposits accumulate enough to plug up a coronary blood vessel, a true heart attack or coronary is the result.

A HEART SAVING PROGRAM

To spare your heart trouble at the outset, the principles of diet are number one on the list. We've seen that weight must be brought down to coincide with your height-weight-frame situation. Consider this series of events in connection with saving your heart:

1. Losing weight decreases the work load on your heart and increases its reserve power.
2. Proper general muscular toning routines insure adequate amounts of vital blood sugar to heart muscle cells and increases the cell's positive metabolism that further increases heart muscle tone.
3. The more heart muscle tone increases, the more extra blood vessels are formed inside the heart muscle itself to bring more vital blood sugar to the cells and to increase the blood reserves.
4. The more blood reserves that develop inside the heart, the

less likely an arterial plug will form (producing a coronary), and if a coronary attack should occur, the more likely you'll survive it without difficulty because of the more efficient healing from the built-up blood reserves.

Take a good look at any of your acquaintances who may have had a coronary between the ages of forty and fifty. How many of them look as though they're making an effort to control their blood sugar? Very few, I'll wager.

WHAT TO DO ABOUT SALT

You've probably heard about, or may even have had to deal with, the question of salt in your diet at one time or another. Why salt? What has this simple compound to do with heart and blood vessel disease? Didn't I say previously that salt is vital to life? Salt *is* vital to life. In heart and blood vessel disease, however, something goes awry with the body's normal handling of salt, and it accumulates in cells and in the blood stream where it becomes a liability to good health. The problem of salt varies with locale. For example, when I practiced in the Arizona desert, I couldn't understand why some of my patients were having difficulty with *too much* salt when I had them on strict diets designed to eliminate salt. I finally realized that the water in Arizona has about 10 times more natural salt in it than does water, say, in Colorado. In Arizona, patients with heart and blood vessel disease sometimes must drink only distilled water.

A Program for Salt Control

Most people could do better with salt control than they do. After the age of forty-five, it's wise to cut down on salt intake as a matter of course whether you may have any sign of heart disease or not. You can do this by observing the following general rules:

1. Stop cooking with salt, baking with salt, and stop adding salt to everything you eat.
2. Use one of the many varieties of salt-substitutes just as you

do with sugar substitutes. These compounds don't taste exactly like the real thing, but they are close enough. They're safe, and they don't react with heart and blood vessels as common table salt may.

3. There is ample salt naturally occurring in many foods so that you needn't fear shorting yourself on salt. Salt is found naturally in meat, fowl, fish, and fresh vegetables in enough quantities to furnish your system with ample salt if these foods are eaten in usual quantities.

HEART STRAIN—IS IT POSSIBLE?

Given good control over blood sugar levels, it's difficult to strain your heart. If blood sugar control is neglected, then certainly the heart can be damaged.

But what of the heart that has already sustained damage? Can it be dealt with like any other heart? Is there hope for the damaged heart? The answer is most certainly YES! You can maintain all the factors for good blood sugar control even if you've already had a coronary. The case that follows is an excellent example of what I mean.

How a Middle-Aged Accountant Coped with a Heart Attack

Harry was 48 years old when he had his first coronary attack. He was of short, stocky stature and about 45 pounds overweight. He is an accountant for a large company that has frequent audits from the government, as well as from various securities people, and it was during one such encounter that Harry had a heart attack. He spent the usual three weeks in the hospital followed by six weeks recuperating at home. There were no complications, and Harry's heart healed well. He was found to be physically well otherwise during his stay in the hospital.

But Harry was of a temperament that allowed this temporary setback to disturb him psychologically. He became extremely fearful of anything that smacked of physical exercise following his recovery. He wouldn't, as a matter of fact, leave his house other than to go out on the front porch. He was afraid the exertion might produce another attack which would be fatal. He was fully convinced that the "strain" from overwork and anxiety at his job caused his heart trouble.

I had a very difficult time trying to talk Harry out of his notions regarding heart trouble, and I've noticed this difficulty in many patients before and after Harry's dilemma. Eventually, I was able to convince Harry that it was all the things that *preceded* his heart attack—his overweight condition, his flabby muscles, in other words, his poor blood sugar control—that caused it. When he accepted this, I went to the tedious second stage—that of trying to convince him that he was *not* a so-called "cardiac cripple" even though he had sustained damage to his heart. The man was almost in a panic. He fought me all the way, insisting that to do anything other than spend his remaining years in a wheel chair was the height of folly. "You don't know, doc," he said, "You never had one like I did!" At this point, I got a little annoyed with Harry. I told him that the only reason that I probably didn't have a coronary was that I was fortunate enough to know how to prevent it, and that I thought his attitude of "I'm the one who's sick" was a little childish for a man his age and intelligence.

This shocked Harry. There followed talk about another doctor, a real specialist in cardiology (heart disease), and so on. I told him I thought this was a great idea. So in a few days, I gave Harry the names of some heart specialists, he selected one, and I discussed Harry's case with the specialist and gave him all of Harry's records and EKG's.

Harry was finally convinced that he need not become an invalid. His specialist told him that if he did, he was a bigger fool than he thought, and that he should listen to well-intended advice and stop feeling sorry for himself. Harry took his advice. He learned that nature has effective ways of letting him know when he was approaching too much exercise, and for the next six months, Harry began to live again. He took long walks, cut down his weight, and began to use good diet sense by cutting out fats, grease, and fried food. He lowered his intake of eggs, baked goods, and sweets. He switched to skim milk and margarine. He ate in a relaxed atmosphere, even though the air was charged with emotional stress at work. He had snacks between meals and drastically cut down on alcohol, coffee, and smoking.

Within the six-month period, Harry was able to resume all his former physical activity. Of course, this wasn't much for Harry, but it was at least a step in the right direction. He began to *cautiously* try a simple exercise routine before bedtime. This routine didn't include sit-ups or any "heavy" exercises, but started with some simple isometrics. When he found he could do these handily and without trouble, he added, *slowly*, some calisthenics. He started with squats and side-bends. When he found he could do these without ill-effect, he slowly added some jogging, usually in the mornings. He didn't try to set records with distance or speed, he just took a slow, easy jogging pace, and when he felt a little winded, he changed to a slow walk. Within two months, he found he could even do some of the more vigorous exercises like push-ups.

The point with this case is that a damaged heart *can* heal and it *can* function well again and usually does. There are, of course, people who have more serious damage with an acute coronary attack, but the doctor in charge of the case can advise of this and set the appropriate limits on exercise. These limits may or may not need to be *permanently* imposed. The passage of time generally allows more and more physical exertion.

BIRTH DEFECTS AND THE HEART

Sometimes nature goofs. She is not always careful as far as the heart is concerned; in fact, there may be a defect somewhere within the heart. When this used to happen just a generation ago, it was regarded as a tragedy. Now, almost every congenital heart defect has come under the corrective scalpel of the heart surgeon. Defects in the heart fall under the following categories:

DEFECTS IN THE HEART WALLS. As a baby develops in the womb, the heart goes through many phases. One of these phases produces a communication through the walls separating the two auricles (upper chambers) and through the wall separating the two ventricles (lower chambers). These holes normally close before birth. Sometimes, they don't. Such persistent defects are called septal (wall) defects. They can be closed surgically and with excellent results.

DEFECTS IN VALVES. Sometimes there is a failure to develop in one of the four valves in the heart. When this happens, the normal openings between the chambers and the great vessels fail to open and close at the proper times. The defective valves can be surgically repaired or even entirely replaced, if necessary. The results are generally quite good.

DEFECTS IN GREAT VESSELS. The great vessels leading to the heart can sometimes be malformed, or nature accidentally hooks one of them to the wrong chamber. The large veins carrying freshly oxygenated blood to the heart, the large arteries carrying blood to the lungs and the aorta, the large artery that carries blood from the left ventricle to all places of the body, can all be involved. Most such abnormalities can be corrected surgically today. At least, the defect can be helped to such an extent that the person needn't become a cardiac cripple.

Thus in our amazing technical age, there aren't any birth defects in the heart that can't be repaired! This is truly an amazing advance when you stop to think about it.

THE ONCE DREADED RHEUMATIC HEART

Rheumatic heart disease is by far the most common of all heart afflictions. It is this disease that causes more than 75 per cent of all the "murmurs" and "leakages" of the human heart. We're now seeing a gradual decline in this once dreaded crippler. Rheumatic heart disease is a strange bird among heart diseases because, basically, it's caused by the secondary effects of a bacterial infection—an infection by a special bug known as the streptococcus. Streptococcus infection, or "strep" as it's commonly called, is the bug responsible for the majority of septic sore throats in youngsters. It's the bug that causes tonsilitis, pharnygitis, ear infections, and scarlet fever. Only a small percentage of those with strep infection, usually young people, but some adults, actually have acute rheumatic fever as an aftermath of such infections, but because the infections are so common, the number of people with rheumatic fever have been considerable.

Rheumatic fever generally occurs about two or three months

following strep throat or scarlet fever. It starts suddenly with fever, hot swollen tender joints, and a generalized "rocky" feeling such as the flu might give. The joints involved may be a left knee, then a right elbow, then a left hip, and finally, the fingers of the right hand. In other words, the disease causes a "migrating" acute arthritis. When the disease leaves the joints, it can begin to affect the heart. When this happens, the heart rate speeds up, there is fever again, and the inside lining of the heart chambers may be inflamed.

All this isn't caused from the strep infection itself, but rather by a hypersensitive (allergic) state that sets in as a result of a patient being allergic to parts of the bacteria itself. It's the antibodies to the protein in these bugs that cause all the damage. Somehow, and it's never been too clear how, strep bugs are able to "fool" the body's antibodies into thinking that certain cells in the joints and heart are the strep bugs themselves. As a result, the "fooled" antibodies attack these cells with all the gusto they would were these cells strep bugs themselves!

The aftermath of all this is that the valves inside the heart chambers may be severely damaged. This causes "leaks" and murmurs, and may incapacitate the patient's heart. The valves most commonly involved are the ones between the left ventricle and auricle and between the left ventricle and the aorta.

No longer need a patient with this type of valve damage be an invalid for the rest of his life, however. Surgery, as with the congenital heart diseases, can repair or replace the damaged valve.

If you have a damaged valve from rheumatic fever, the first thing to determine is whether the valve is damaged severely enough to produce symptoms. Your doctor probably already knows what the story is and can advise you on such things as diet and physical exertion. If you must curtail certain activities, you may be a candidate for heart surgery. Your doctor can see that you receive the necessary referral, if this seems indicated.

It certainly follows that exercise routines need to be closely watched by you and your doctor if you've had rheumatic fever in the past. If there is doubt, seek expert advice *before* you attempt strenuous exercise.

WHAT TO DO ABOUT HIGH BLOOD PRESSURE

High blood pressure, or hypertension, is a symptom of a disease state of the organism in which, for a variety of reasons, the arteries aren't as flexible as they should be. Whenever a blood vessel, especially an artery, becomes rigid, the pressure on the blood inside it rises.

Many people have formed the idea that it's the heart that causes high blood pressure. This notion is wrong. The heart is *affected* by high blood pressure, but it doesn't *cause* it. The basic fault lies in the arteries throughout the system.

Think of high blood pressure in this way: Notice the water coming out the end of a garden hose nozzle—it's under a great deal more pressure than the water coming out of the spigot to which the hose attaches, right? This is because you've added *resistance* beyond the spigot. Increased resistance causes increased pressure. It's the same with your arteries. If the resistance of the muscular artery tubing is increased, the pressure will go up because the heart must pump harder to get the blood through the stiffer tubing. To make matters worse, once the resistance inside the artery goes up and blood pressure begins to rise, the increased pressure, itself, tends to make the artery more rigid over a period of time, and there is a vicious circle set up that increases the problem if something isn't done to interrupt it.

Hypertension and Nervousness

There are sometimes "gray areas" between true hypertension and a normal situation. An example is a patient I saw recently whose blood pressure was 168/108 when I first examined him. If I were to have taken this first reading as the usual one for him, I would have had to conclude that he did, indeed, have high blood pressure. The usual critical level for sustained blood pressure is about 150/100. If the blood pressure is below this figure *consistently*, there is *no* hypertension. If it's *consistently* above this level, then hypertension does exist and must be dealt with.

The patient just referred to was a highly nervous man in his mid-thirties. He had always known good health and looked the picture of good physical condition at the time of his examination. A week later, I recorded his pressure again and it was 126/82— perfectly normal. And it stayed that way over a period of the next two weeks. It wasn't until he became emotionally involved again, some weeks later, that his pressure again exceeded the critical level. This man does *not* have hypertension, but merely has a nervous system that pushes his pressure up on occasion. These elevations will never cause the patient damage so long as it comes back down to normal again, as I expect it will.

BLOOD PRESSURE RECORDING SYSTEM

You may be somewhat puzzled by the two figures always mentioned regarding blood pressure. The first figure, the one always given *above* the line (the 168 in the case just mentioned), represents the pressure during the beat of the two heart ventricles. This figure is called the *systolic* pressure. The second figure, the one given below the line (the 108 in the case just mentioned), represents the pressure inside the artery during the relaxed phase of the heart beat—when the ventricles are filling up with blood from the auricles.

It's the figure below the line, the *diastolic* pressure as its called, that is by far the most important of the two. Everybody's *systolic* blood pressure goes up during exercise, climbing stairs, jogging, etc. Yours, mine and everybody else's does—it's natural and normal for it to do so. However, rarely does anyone's *diastolic* blood pressure rise above the 100 mark even during strenuous exercise unless there's something wrong with those arteries. The point to remember here is that if only your *systolic* pressure is elevated at any given measurement, you don't have much to worry about. If your *diastolic* pressure is over the critical mark consistently, even if the *systolic* pressure is fairly normal, you must assume trouble and begin to correct it.

When I'm faced with a blood pressure that's consistently close to 150/100 on repeated determinations, I take a close look, as I did recently with a middle-aged woman, to see how well the patient has attended to his blood sugar levels as reflected in such things as height-weight-frame ratio, diet, muscle tone, and so on. This particular lady had not been properly schooled in blood sugar regulation. She was sixty pounds overweight with regard to her height and frame, she was flabby and soft of muscle and had little in the way of discipline and will power. With this woman, reduction of weight, restriction of salt, and a course in muscle toning reduced her pressure to acceptable levels. Her blood pressure has never exceeded 130/86 since starting this routine.

SALT AGAIN. There are certain changes that take place in the kidneys that start other changes during high blood pressure. The changes that are produced cause the organism to handle the elimination of excess salt very poorly. The salt collects in the tissues in excess amounts; that is, salt that's not really needed after the cells have all they need. When excess salt accumulates in tissues, it causes the condition commonly known as "dropsy." Dropsy occurs when your ankles, lower legs, thighs, and sometimes even your upper extremities swell up with fluid. When this happens, you can press the swollen areas with your finger and a "dent" is left in the skin. This "dent" indicates you have too much salt in your system and that you must eliminate it.

If salt in excess collects in tissues, it acts like a sponge. And like a sponge, it attracts water into the tissues. Most people I've observed eat far too much salt. It's a good idea to cut down on salt, as I've mentioned before, after the age of forty-five or so. If high blood pressure enters the picture, salt elimination *is a must*. This is why the usual first drug treatment for high blood pressure is one that stimulates your kidneys to eliminate excess fluid, therefore, excess salt. In an appendix at the end of this book is an example of how to select a diet that's salt poor, or even salt free if required. Remember, you'll get enough vital salt through protein foods and vegetables.

HIGH BLOOD PRESSURE IS PREVENTABLE

Although there are a few rare diseases that can cause high blood pressure as part of their course, 95 per cent of it can be prevented. And it's not too late to start even if you may already have an elevated pressure!

Strange as it may seem, doctors don't particularly like to nag about weight to their patients. It's just that they know what happens when excess weight is present. High blood pressure is only one of a multitude of diseases, as you've already learned, that may result merely from the overweight factor. Consider these steps in the development of blood pressure trouble:

A Case History of Avoidable Heart Trouble

1. Patient well until age thirty-five. Began to put on weight until age forty, when weight was thirty pounds over the height-frame levels.
2. Patient used to be active. Now, at age forty-one, has better job, activity reduced, beginning to worry about children's college education, and other problems of "better living."
3. Routine check at age forty-two shows blood pressure 136/90. Assured "everything O.K." Nothing said about eating, drinking, smoking, physical activity, or worry habits.
4. Another check at age forty-four shows pressure 146/96. *Still nothing done about blood sugar level habits.*
5. At age fifty, spouse has gone to work to support college tuition for children, total weight gain of 45 pounds has occurred, smoking increased to two packs a day, drinking on upswing, outside physical activity has reduced to nothing.
6. Pressure is now 164/110 and steady at this figure. Patient having angina of effort (heart pain on exertion), headaches, and vision trouble. All this and more could have been prevented. Steps could have been started between stages 1 and 2. If they had, patient would have been well today. Instead, he is recovering from a stroke.

These stages are taken from a case history. It happened, and it's continuing to happen every day of the year, year in and year out. *You* can bring a stop to it if you desire. Start now to preserve your heart and blood vessels by remembering the following rules:

WEIGHT. Get yourself in line with the tables in Chapter 3. Don't wait until next week to start—now is the time! If you already have high blood pressure and you know you're overweight, save yourself a stroke and lose those pounds!

WORRY. Nerves do play a vital role in high blood pressure disease. Get them under control *now*. Start getting that excess mental energy drained off by starting your physical routines *today!* Don't wait until next week. If you already have high blood pressure and are soft and flabby, start your routines slowly and with caution, but start. If you have symptoms, you're overdoing it. Reduce the number of exercises and stop straining so hard, but keep them up.

SMOKING. Although no one ever has proven that smoking *causes* high blood pressure, it invariably makes an existing high blood pressure worse. Cut smoking by 75 per cent today.

If you have trouble with any of the foregoing principles, utilize what you've learned about mind control. Use it to help you diet, to help you start exercise schedules and stick to them, use it to help you resolve those perplexing mental conflicts that beset your life, and use it to concentrate on relaxation of all your blood vessel walls when you retire at night—the muscles that surround the arteries, remember, are under nerve control. Use this knowledge to help you out of what could be serious trouble later!

NOT WHERE, BUT *HOW* YOU LIVE IS THE IMPORTANT THING

You may have noticed that the mode of life—the stressful things —played an important part in the cases presented in this section. They play a part in everybody's life. There's no escaping life's problems, so the thing to do is to come to grips with all of them. There is no such thing as an insoluble problem. Some of them may seem so, but it's only because the possibilities of settlement haven't been completely worked out that they appear to be insurmountable. In order of importance, I'd say the following categories deserved immediate attention in turn: Marriage, Work and Self.

MARRIAGE. I recently took care of a man whose marriage had been on the rocks for five years or longer, but nothing had been resolved. He and his wife hadn't worked out the problems. His blood pressure was up. He needed blood sugar control badly, but this problem kept him from being able to free his mind to do anything about it. When things went from bad to worse, both he and his wife saw less of each other. Soon things got bad with the youngsters at home. The patient's blood pressure climbed. This couple literally had to be forced to a solution which was the usual strife with the lawyers, strife with the kids, and continuing strife with alimony.

This kind of struggle is never worthwhile. Marriage problems can be solved or dissolved rather early in the game, if the people involved are interested. If you have such problems, I suggest you get to their source as quickly as possible. Most find that the trouble lies with both partners—I've never seen it one-sided, though I've been approached by both partners singly hundreds of times where the conversation began with, "It's my wife's (husband's) fault, doctor . . . ." If I'd listened to the first partner's story, I'd have fallen into a common trap. I never draw conclusions until *all* parties are heard from in such questions.

Face it. For all your partner's faults, don't you have just one or two? If so, at least you're honest. The point is, until you've corrected them so that you're perfect, don't moan too loudly about your spouse.

WORK. Your boss may well be "impossible." That does not indicate that you need to lose sleep over it, but I know many who do. And they work up a high head of steam in doing so. The mark of maturity is the man who can say, "I accept you for what you are, but I'm not playing your game."

Deadlines raise blood pressure. People who work under the constant threat and pressure of a deadline of any kind are excellent candidates for high blood pressure and heart attacks. You can tolerate deadlines *if you have good blood sugar control.* If not, you'd better get that way if you're working under conditions where time-production is important. If you've already acquired heart disease or high blood pressure, the only answer may be to change jobs so that this factor of deadline isn't present.

Why a Patient Changed Jobs

The patient I took care of with such a problem was in the tax accounting business. He had a severe heart attack at age fifty-two.

It was so severe that he was never able to resume good blood sugar control—he couldn't strain physically for exercise routines. He changed jobs, and at least has not had a recurrent attack. He keeps accounting books for a small manufacturer now, and has no deadlines to meet.

SELF. Some people with heart and blood vessel disease are their own worst enemy. They're afraid or they're angry or they're over-rated.

I knew a woman who was so afraid of failing as a mother and a wife of a high-powered executive that she developed high blood pressure. Another man was so frustrated at his supposed sorry plight in life that his subsequent anger caused him high blood pressure. Yet another woman was so incensed with her superiority over her male counterparts in the business world that she drove herself to the top of her field, and to severe hypertension.

What all these cases have in common are problems with themselves as human beings. Without going into all the complicated Freudian analytic background theory, it can be said of these people that they haven't yet discovered themselves; they haven't come to terms with life and put themselves into a rational place in the scheme of things. Most people who don't find their "place" by the time they're thirty or forty years old generally end up with trouble. Often, the problem lodges itself in the cardiovascular system.

This is why Chapter 5 is so important, and why I recommend to many patients that they ask themselves the simple question, "Why?" Why am I breaking my neck for something that really isn't worth it? Why am I afraid of losing, or of failing? Can I really win them all? Why am I depressed from always being angry? Am I getting rid of hostility efficiently? Why the hostility, anyway? Are "they" all really that threatening?

It's the answer to such questions, and their smooth solutions, that may mean the difference between health and disease. If you haven't taken stock recently, I suggest you take the time to do so. You may save yourself from blowing a gasket.

ORGAN TRANSPLANTS: A NEW ERA

Recently, in the city in which I live, a man underwent a spectacular piece of surgery. Not only did he have a new heart transplanted into his chest to replace his diseased one, but he also received a new kidney from the same donor at the same surgery! The successes of organ transplant are certainly fantastic. But again, a hundred doors have been opened, each posing unanswered problems. Who decides when a donor (the individual from whose body an organ is removed) is "dead"? If one or more of his organs can be salvaged, isn't it possible that he might be "revived"? What happens in the event a choice must be made as to who gets the benefit of a donor's organs? What of the host of legal implications? Could the families of donors be considered to have certain vested interests in the person receiving such organs? Shall criminals be donors? Or, for that matter, receivers of organ transplants?

These and hundreds of other questions will have to be answered. In any event, it's likely that urgent attention to blood sugar control will be all the more important as we find ourselves thrust headlong into the organ transplant era.

SUMMARY

1. Your heart must be able to perform its duty of pumping blood uninterruptedly day in and day out. The principles of good blood sugar control are perfect guides to keep your heart at peak efficiency.
2. Most heart and blood vessel diseases can be prevented. Careful attention to your height-weight-frame ratios, proper exercise, and proper mind control can be brought into play to prevent and to guide recovery from heart and artery disease.
3. Heart and blood vessel afflictions caused from sources other than your own neglect, such as rheumatic heart disease and birth defects, are now being cured surgically. If any of these conditions stand in the way of your efficient blood sugar con-

trol, you may be able to overcome them. When you do, all the principles discussed thus far will enable you to get your blood sugar levels where they should be for lasting health.

4. Attention to blood sugar levels can prevent high blood pressure. If high blood pressure has already become a factor in your health, use blood sugar principles to help yourself out of this rut.

5. The task of judging the social, moral and philosophical questions raised by organ transplant lies with you, the American public. Be aware of such problems. Don't turn a deaf ear to them because you may eventually need to cope with them, either because you may need such attention yourself or a member of your family may be involved.

8

How to Fight Alcoholism with Blood Sugar Control

Alcoholism is a growing problem in this country. It's hard to find accurate facts and figures on just how big the problem really is, but alcoholics in this country number in the 8–10 million range at this time. This doesn't take into account huge numbers of others who are semi-alcoholics—the ones who aren't quite there yet, but soon will be. I want to discuss this disease with you in relation to its important bearing on low blood sugar.

This chapter will examine the vital part the liver and endocrine glands play in alcoholism, and how blood sugar control can protect you from irreversible alcoholic disease. There are also some "rules of thumb" by which you can tell whether you, or someone in your family, may be an alcoholic or becoming one, and what to do about it if it occurs.

WHAT CAUSES ALCOHOLISM?

Twenty years ago, alcoholism was thought to be simply a bad habit brought on by loose living. A decade or so ago, the thinking changed, and we were told that alcoholism is a disease. Unfortunately, try as they might, scientists and researchers have been unable to tell us just where this disease begins—in what organ or system of organs alcoholism starts. Are the changes found in body organs in people who are already alcoholics causes or effects of too much alcohol? The evidence indicates alcohol produces all kinds of changes in the body and mind, but there's nothing yet to substantiate that a defect in some organ exists that isn't there in people who never took a drink of whiskey in their lives.

Shortly after the "disease" theory on alcoholism started, psychiatrists branded alcoholism a mental illness, caused by the presence of certain personality traits and family troubles during childhood development. The trouble with this explanation is that it doesn't spell out just what these personality traits are, or exactly why thousands of other people who have the "alcoholic personality traits" don't suffer alcoholism. Furthermore, the correction of such personality traits and family abnormalities seems to have little effect on the course of an alcoholic person, nor has it been demonstrated that alcoholism can be prevented if you catch the person with the neurotic personality early enough. To understand better how alcoholism begins, let's take a patient from the beginning of his problem and follow it along.

Case History of an Alcoholic

Al is twenty-five. He has a wife and family, and he holds down a good job. He is not an especially clean-cut, all-American boy, but neither is he a bad citizen, a criminal, or cruel to his family. In fact, Al is a good husband, or at least he has been until recently, when his wife noticed that Al spends more and more time away from home—he's out with the boys on drinking sprees, at poker parties, or just "out." Much as Al knows how his being away from home affects his wife and kids, much as he'd like to stop the growing habit, he can't. He feels powerless to resist that first drink that leads to a second and third, and so on until he ends up on the floor dead drunk.

This is only the beginning of Al's problem, but let's retrace the case. You might reasonably ask, wasn't Al doing a lot of drinking before? Wasn't he the victim of bad company earlier? The answer is "no," he wasn't. Al had the kind of early life and childhood that tens of millions of other people his age have had. He was neither an excellent student nor a poor one. He had the usual advantage of a good home with attentive parents. His education was as good as that of 75 per cent of young men his age. His stint in the Army was clean, and he possessed an honorable discharge. Al married a girl he met while in the Army and they had a good marriage with two kids both normal in all respects. Their marital union had no more nor less than the usual pressures applied to it over the past eight years.

By now, although Al knows what just taking that "first shot" will do to him, he's in the throes of alcoholism: He hides a bottle in the house and nips heavily when his wife isn't around. He takes every advantage of her good nature to spend the evening at a local bar with friends or at their house for a "real bust." He has a couple of drinks in the morning before work, again at noon if he can squeeze in the time, and before coming home to dinner, if he can afford it. And this is where the trouble is brewing: Al has gone through their savings, has borrowed money to support his liquor consumption, and is trying to hold down a second job to add to the depleted funds. Al's wife now begins to get tough. She threatens, cajoles, leaves for mother's a few times (only to return), and finally consults a lawyer. Al promises to go on the wagon, and does for a day or two, but jumps right off at the first opportunity. When she leaves for mother's, Al just goes on a continuous binge and begins to have blackouts at the end of them. And he can't remember anything at all that happened during the two or three days after these black-outs.

Meanwhile, Al's wife has started legal separation procedures and has contacted Al's boss at work who threatened Al with firing. Al hops briefly on the wagon once more, but things get worse. He begins to carouse around with other women on his binges, gets in fights, and acquires a police record. He loses both jobs, his wife and family and has a convulsion while coming off the booze—he ends up in a hospital for five days.

Now you'd think that Al would have had reason enough to shape up long before this. He was threatened with the loss of home and family, he was having frequent mental black-outs, and he was rapidly going broke paying for his liquor. Al isn't stupid, remember. He knows perfectly well what's happening and what's going to happen if he doesn't stop. But he doesn't stop, because he *can't stop*. And, to summarize the events that followed Al's hospitalization with the convulsions, he hasn't stopped yet. His life has settled itself down to periods of long binges alternating with dry periods where he's off alcohol, but his problem is still there. Not even the loss of his family and self-respect has cured him. Even the fact that he's now got irreversible liver damage and is heading for chronic brain damage (and life-time institutionalization, if this happens) hasn't deterred him from his destructive course. Why? He's had help: Alcoholics Anonymous entered the picture when Al's wife threatened divorce. He's been to a psychiatrist recommended by his former boss. And he's been involved in his city's special alcohol program, financed in part by the government. None has helped him for more than a short time. Why?

The reason is that Al is one of the 5 per cent of the population whose body can't handle alcohol in the normal fashion. Why can't Al and others in his boat handle alcohol? Because they have different metabolism than most, and because Al and other alcoholics also have personality problems. Put these two things together—a personality disturbance and a metabolic deficiency—and you have an alcoholic.

This means that there are people in our country equal in number to all the known alcoholics who are potential alcoholics. These represent people who have the same metabolic disturbance Al has, but they aren't driven to drink by personality problems. They'll never know alcoholism because they have no special reason to become alcoholics. This is also why there are millions of people in the country with personality difficulties similar to all the Al's who are alcoholics, but who don't become alcoholics because they *can stop drinking* after the first few shots—they don't have a metabolic defect.

We see here, again, an example of the train I drew in discussing the question of arthritis. You have two distinct entities which, if they occur together, make a condition; if either occurs without the other, you don't have the condition.

THE ALCOHOLIC PERSONALITY

What was wrong in Al's case? Why did he have to drink? Like most others in the same situation, Al was, or felt like he was, dominated by something outside himself that he couldn't control or that was forever beyond his control. This feeling in the personality of drinkers is rather constant. The "force" or "domineering factor" can be a mother, a father, a mother-in-law, a personal tragedy or failure, or even a "cruel world."

THE ALCOHOL METABOLIC DEFECT

The other side of the alcohol coin, the metabolic side, is interesting because it has to do with the way your body burns sugar.

Recall that the pancreas produces insulin, and insulin is what enables the trillions of cells to be able to use sugar for their energy. Recall that the adrenal glands stimulate the liver to release stored sugar, and that they prod the liver into synthesizing sugar from other sources if sugar isn't available in quantities large enough to meet the demand of the cells. Recall also that the pituitary gland, the master endocrine gland, controls the action of both these glands, and is, itself, under the influence of brain hormones and nerve control.

What Happens When a Person Takes a Drink

If a person with *normal* metabolism takes a drink, the following events occur:

1. Alcohol absorbed into bloodstream—oxidized (burned) by certain enzymes in the liver.
2. Before alcohol is completely burned by liver enzymes, it goes to cells where it slows down all metabolism going on there, including that of sugar.
3. In the pancreas, alcohol stimulates excess insulin by blocking the usual "checks" on such excess.
4. Blood sugar drops somewhat by excess insulin. Liver produces more sugar.
5. Cells in the brain increase their demand for sugar because of (4). This demand is met by the liver.

In the alcoholic, something happens to disrupt the above flow of events. Something is out of adjustment! That "something" goes like this:

1. The cells of the brain account for up to 25 per cent of the total sugar metabolism of the body. Impairment of this supply, even for a matter of minutes, is a serious situation. I've already discussed with you some of the elaborate ways nature has provided for emergencies in this regard.
2. Alcoholic takes a drink. He *craves* his first few drinks because something in his metabolism fails to do the job with the sugar levels in the cells of his brain.
3. The initial alcohol he takes satisfied *for the moment* his brain cells' urgent call for sugar, because alcohol is burned somewhat like sugar. But this doesn't last long because alcohol then *depresses* the blood sugar levels to an even greater degree than they were.
4. The alcoholic craves more alcohol in an attempt to correct this hypoglycemic (low blood sugar) state. The vicious circle continues: The brain cells demand more alcohol to replace the lack of sugar. Hence, the alcohol crave.

It's unfortunate that no one knows precisely where this defect in metabolism lies. It may be primarily in the liver. Or in the adrenal glands. Or it may be in the pituitary master gland. But it's known that it does exist. And, in keeping with the premise raised earlier in the book, it really doesn't matter at this point where the defect lies. *Low blood sugar levels, and with it, low brain cell sugar levels, can be prevented!*

THE EFFECTS OF PROLONGED ALCOHOL EXCESS

You can now appreciate some of the problems of an alcoholic. Here's a person with a particular personality and with a metabolic defect that actually makes his brain cells demand more alcohol at the expense of his total physical health! Another example of how important nature deems the continuous function of the brain cells as the prime objective in the human organism.

CARBOHYDRATE METABOLISM. The prolonged intake of excess alcohol begins to take its physical and mental toll in the form of altered burning of energy. After a time, not only do the brain cells come to crave alcohol, but all the rest of the cells as well. The body chemistry of an alcoholic is entirely changed from one of a system that burns sugar as the sole source of energy to one that burns alcohol as the chief source of its energy. The lack of carbohydrates in an alcoholic has its first effect in the way his body handles fat.

Fat is normally deposited around muscles and in the abdominal cavity, as I've mentioned before. In the alcoholic, fat is improperly handled and is deposited directly in the liver. The reason is that the liver needs the fat to produce energy since carbohydrate is no longer available in the alcoholic. Remember, the fat can be burned, though inefficiently, as energy.

The trouble with this liver "depot" of fat in an alcoholic is that the sheer bulk of this deposited fat begins to slow the liver down in its other function. An example of a vital liver function that's disrupted by the presence of all this fat is the manufacture of vital proteins. When this happens, the body loses protein from muscle tissue. This is why long standing alcoholics are thin and starved looking. Their livers can't make enough protein.

To review again the body's protein manufacturing system: If need be, the body can make protein from carbohydrate. There being a shortage of carbohydrate, the body craves even more alcohol for this manufacture. More of the vicious circle! After a certain time, the body's ability to use carbohydrate, even when it's furnished in adequate amounts in the diet, becomes impaired. This is a point of no return for an alcoholic, because his body has been too much altered by his excesses. This emphasizes the serious need for *prevention* in alcoholism.

LIVER DAMAGE. As the liver sustains more and more injury from alcoholism, it begins to enlarge in an attempt to keep up with its work. I've seen livers reach such size in chronic alcoholics that it occupied the entire abdomen! At a certain stage in this enlargement, other changes than carbohydrate and protein metabolism take place. One of the first things that happens is that the large blood vessels that supply the liver with blood become blocked off because of the huge size of the organ and because as liver cells are destroyed, scarring takes place that prevents blood from flowing through the liver. When these blood vessels are blocked, the body has no alternative but to bypass the liver. When this happens, the blood vessels inside the tube leading from the mouth to the stomach (esophagus) become hugely engorged (they aren't used to carrying this extra load of blood) and may burst, causing profuse hemorrhage. This is why some alcoholics suddenly vomit blood.

Also as the liver enlarges, the bile formed in liver cells finds no way to get out and into the gall bladder. Bile is backed up in the blood stream and jaundice results. Jaundice occurs when the skin turns yellow. Bile, remember, is necessary in the digestive process inside the intestine. If there's no way for bile to get into the intestine, digestion is seriously impaired and the nutrition status, already compromised by the effect of carbohydrate and protein shortage, worsens. If food that's eaten can't be digested, it's presence will hardly help the person!

CIRRHOSIS. With the death of hundreds of liver cells increasing with every alcoholic binge, the ultimate blow to the alcoholic liver is a condition known as cirrhosis (pronounced: seerohsis). This is another irreversible situation in which so many liver cells have been killed that there is permanent liver disease. Jaundice (yellow skin) may be the first clue to cirrhosis. Severe pain and nausea and vomiting may be another. A downhill course with general health is the rule. Weight is lost, appetite is lost, strength and vitality is lost, a young man may appear thirty years older than his actual age and death may result, if not enough normal cells remain to carry out the multiple functions the liver provides.

The advent of cirrhosis, however, need not spell doom. If cirrhosis has already entered the picture, nature will respond to help. The help consists of, first and foremost, stopping the death of liver cells from this point on—*no more alcohol in any form whatever!* The second rule is *the intake of adequate carbohydrate.* At this point, the liver is in a turmoil. It needs all the protection it can get so that all its former functions can return to near normal. Such protection is forthcoming in the form of increased carbohydrate in the diet because carbohydrate reverses the low blood sugar situation and helps restore fat and protein metabolism to normal. Normal fat metabolism releases the liver from having to use vital proteins for energy so it can devote its attention to the production of protein for muscle, enzyme, and endocrine secretions. In short, you may see once again, as throughout this book, the basic wisdom of the tenets of adequate blood sugar maintenance! And what starting this basic blood sugar maintenance program can do *even when severe disease has entered the picture as in diabetes or alcoholism.*

WHEN IS A PERSON AN ALCOHOLIC?

Most people who drink heavily will deny that they are an alcoholic. The more they drink, the more definite will be their denial. One of the first obstacles in any alcohol treatment center is convincing patients that they are, indeed, alcoholics! If they can't or won't accept the fact that they are, treatment fails at the outset.

There are many fancy classifications of alcoholism. A variety of complicated methods have been proposed for detecting an alcoholic. In my opinion, there is a very simple way to tell if you're headed for trouble with alcohol!

1. When you drink, you should be able and willing to have one or two in the evening after work without desire for more.
2. At a gathering or party, three or four drinks in the course of the evening should be your natural habit.
3. During the day, there should be no desire whatever for a drink.
4. You should be perfectly at ease watching others on their way to alcohol oblivion without feeling the slightest remorse yourself.
5. If you've ever had a hangover (and most people who have ever taken alcohol have), the complete loathing and rejection of the feeling a hangover brings should convince you that another one is out of the question.

If your alcohol pattern doesn't fit this guide, you're either on the way or have arrived at alcoholism!

All sorts of excuses will now come up for not fitting into this pattern with alcohol. Everything from the voice inside that says "pay no attention"—what do they know—to laughing at the whole ridiculous thing—"nobody's going to tell me when or how much I'm going to drink." Remember my discussion of the personality of the alcoholic. There are a hundred reasons why you may want to drink excessively. Some of them may seem quite valid and convincing. But none of them will protect your liver from damage or your brain from deteriorating. The one thing that *will* protect you is the frank, unfettered-by-excuse admission *to yourself* that you've got a problem. You're now ready to do something about the situation.

It's that *first drink* for an alcoholic that's fatal. Even if you're only on the way to being an alcoholic and you recognize it, *you must condition yourself that any first drink will be your eventual undoing!*

There's no such thing as "just one for the road," or one to relax with at night. The only answer is *stop drinking*. The following rules will help in this process:

1. Realize that part of the problem is the personality make-up and part is a *chronic low blood sugar situation* in the body.

   A. You must learn to avoid all situations that drive you to the first drink. If it's your mother-in-law or your husband that does it, admit it. Face the problem with the others concerned—talk it over and begin to try to straighten out the difficulties so they can become a thing of the past. Don't just run away from them and bury your discomfort in liquor. To repeat an example I've used before, this is like treating the rash on the skin caused by typhoid fever—you're just curing the skin and leaving the disease to run its course.

   B. *Start today to correct the low blood sugar situation.* That craving for the first drink means that your *blood sugar levels are low, that your capacity for sugar reserves is low,* and that your brain cells, the first to detect low sugar, are calling for something—alcohol is most nearly like sugar in metabolism. If you take that first drink, you won't be able to stop. *Take carbohydrate instead.* This is one situation in which pure sugar may be preferable to nothing at all, and most certainly preferable to alcohol! At this moment of craving, a soft cola drink, a candy bar, piece of pastry, or a rich dessert of any kind is necessary. Drink a malted milk or milk shake or eat a sandwich. *Do not take stimulants of any kind* (coffee, tea, drugs, etc.) *as this will make the craving worse!*

Then simply follow the rules of diet already outlined in Chapter 3.

2. You already know that physical activity increases the demand on your sugar reserves. Ordinarily, muscular exertion is an excellent way to head off cravings or desires of any kind. With alcoholism, however, the restoration of normal blood sugar comes first—replenish sugar initially. An hour or two later, indulge in strenuous physical activity, then replace that blood sugar *again when you're through*.

3. Mind control must be mastered in alcoholism if you expect results. If you skimmed through Chapter 5 of the book, *read it carefully* two or three more times. Memorize it. And put it to work for your problems. You can utilize mind control in new habit formations to replace alcohol. You can use it in all phases of blood sugar control habits and routines. You can use it to probe personality problems that plague you and drive you into the bar down the street. You can use it to condition your mind to crave other things than alcohol—substances like carbohydrate, physical activity, or intellectual pursuits that aren't harmful and actually help you overcome the urge to drink and your dependence on alcohol. And you can use it to come to grips with those things in your life that have forced you to the bottle in the first place: what to do about the people who dominate you; the people you don't get along with; the people who bring out the worst in you and cause you to run to the bottle.

4. Recognize and face the need for help. Get medical help for your health that may have already been affected by alcohol and mental help for the personality problems that may elude your search for a solution for them. Seek advice from anyone you respect about your problems at work,

home, and play that may have any bearing on your alcoholic excess.

Admitting that you need help is hard. It's quite a blow to your prestige to admit to someone, especially a friend, that alcohol is a problem. *But you need that very friendship to help you.* Ask for it today!

A look at alcoholics in treatment at various centers will show that for every woman in treatment there are three or four men. This, I believe, reflects some interesting points.

First, it's well known that women have more efficient body chemistry than men. And they have more will power. I believe, too, that women have more success on their own at stopping the alcohol habit than men. This doesn't necessarily mean that more men have an alcoholic problem than women. It's just that women have a better success rate with alcohol than men.

Hazel, a woman in her forties, is an example of what I mean. Hazel had been slipping into alcoholism over a period of ten years. She was married, but had no children. She was finally divorced by her husband. She developed early cirrhosis. Her problem became so bad that she was finishing at least a fifth of vodka a day, sometimes for two or three weeks running. Such binges were invariably followed by black-outs during which she couldn't remember anything that occurred during her binges. One day, following a particularly long binge, she had the DT's—Delerium tremens—a condition that causes an alcoholic to see and hear things that aren't actually there. These are hallucinations similar to those psychotic people have. The DT's were the turning point for Hazel.

She sought help from a local alcohol program in which she was admitted to a treatment center as a patient for a week—in a halfway house for a week—and an out-patient for three weeks. During this time, she was able to reduce her severe weight problem by about thirty pounds, start a graduated exercise routine every day, and learn about her personality.

Hazel had wanted to become a nurse. She even entertained the idea of going into medicine (she would have made an excellent doctor—she had brains, compassion, and interest in people). Her desires, however, were continually thwarted by an almost tyrannical step-father who dominated her life with an iron fist. Thus she was unable to realize her ambition in nursing or medicine.

She found that one drink followed another, and that soon, she was unable to resist a state of drunkenness so deep she passed out. She was delivered in this state many times to the local city general hospital.

Hazel had both the personality and biochemistry for the ravages of alcoholism. At the treatment center, it was determined that her liver disease was not yet irreversible, so that she still had the potential of good health if she could get her drinking under control. This, the treatment program helped her to do. While in the program, Hazel began to be acutely aware of the serious effects of alcohol on others in the program. At the termination of her treatment, and with good control over her chemistry and personality, she applied for a job on the staff at the treatment center. At the present time, Hazel is one of the top members of the treatment staff at the institution. She hasn't touched liquor in any form for ten years, and most likely never will. She is cured. And more than that, she has fulfilled her childhood desire to be of tangible service to fellow human beings with problems of mind and body. Hazel has overcome both the chemistry and personality deficits in the problem of alcoholism.

Today, industry is well aware of the problems of alcohol among their employees from the executive level down to the janitor. Industry knows that billions of dollars in lost production and inefficiency are lost every year because of alcohol. There are fields of opportunity open and begging for people to help with such problems. You might consider one of them if you're really interested in helping someone out of the rut of alcoholism.

Try not to look down your nose at the next drunken person you see. He has a serious problem. Try not to avoid the next drunk you see at a party. He needs help badly. Try to understand the ramifications of the alcoholic and his multiple troubles. You might even find it interesting enough to consider as an avocation or something to do when you're retired. You won't regret becoming involved in it.

SUMMARY

1. Alcoholism is an ever-increasing problem in this country. The roots of an alcoholic's problem go deeply into his body chemistry and his personality. The chemical defect is low blood sugar. The

personality defect is over-domination by anything "outside" himself.

2. The brain cells of an alcoholic are starved for sugar. Not getting this vital energy substance in sufficient quantities, brain cells utilize the burning of alcohol as a poor, but only, alternative substitute. The first drink calls for more and more as a result of the vicious circle set up by the first drink.

3. Chronic alcoholism causes disturbances in carbohydrate, fat, and finally, protein metabolism in the body. These disturbances in turn cause disease, primarily in the liver and brain, but if prolonged, in virtually every organ in the body. Usually, these disturbing processes can be reversed. The reversal *always* depends upon following the principles of good blood sugar control as outlined in this book.

4. Alcoholism seriously affects virtually all industry as well as any enterprise that depends on efficient function of the human mind and body for its success. The accidental deaths and injuries caused directly or indirectly by the problem of alcoholism have become a major public health consideration.

5. You can overcome alcoholism in yourself and in others by facing its symptoms and by adhering to the principles of good blood sugar control both in preventing and treating alcoholism.

9

How to Mobilize Your Blood Sugar Defenses
When Disease Strikes

What can I do when disease strikes? You've undoubtedly asked yourself this question numerous times. In this chapter, I want to discuss disease with you and point out some things you can do if you're the unfortunate victim of disease, or if you haven't had to come to grips with disease states, what you can do to prevent them.

I shall discuss the way to deal with emphysema, asthma, and stomach ulcers. I'll talk about these first, not because I think they are the most serious, but because they're the most common.

I'll discuss diseases of the intestinal tract, kidneys, and rheumatism because they're not only common, but a lot of folk lore exists about where these diseases come from and what to do about them once they're on the scene. And I'll talk about surgery—the relation of surgical success to blood sugar levels and how to come through with flying colors.

All disease, no exceptions, either can be prevented by good habits of blood sugar control or made much less serious. You've already seen this concerning your heart and blood vessels and alcoholism. Now I'll show you what you can do with a wide variety of disease with blood sugar control.

HOW TO COPE WITH EMPHYSEMA

Emphysema is a lung disease. As I've already pointed out, emphysema affects those tiny grape-like clusters of air sacs where the oxygen is absorbed into your blood stream and carbon dioxide (the waste from sugar burning) passes out. Both these products are gasses. They pass through the unbelievably thin air-sac walls by their own pressure. If anything happens to the walls of these tiny air sacs, trouble occurs!

Emphysema causes the opposite effect of asthma—instead of the air sacs being constricted as in asthma, making it difficult to get air into your lungs—in emphysema, the sacs are greatly expanded, ballooned out. They've lost their elasticity. They can't squeeze down. As a consequence, the job of getting air out is what is made difficult.

CAUSES. There are two main types of emphysema. One results from the simple process of aging—if a person lives long enough, he will have a certain amount of emphysema change in his lungs. The other is the acquired type—the type that begins much too early in life to be caused by aging, though you might regard it as a kind of premature aging process. What starts this type of emphysema? Too much cigarette smoking is probably the most common cause. Working at a job that causes you to breathe irritating substances is probably the second most common cause.

Some lungs seem more susceptible to emphysema than do others, but underlying most every case of emphysema is—the irritation factor. It follows that if you have or are in the process of getting emphysema, the first thing you're going to have to do is to block the irritating factor—to stop breathing in the things that irritate those air sacs and cause them to lose their ability to be flexible.

SYMPTOMS. The first symptom of this disease can be hard to spot, but you can if you're alert. You find yourself running short of breath while doing physical activities that wouldn't have bothered you a year or so ago. You walk a block or two and you're puffing and short-winded—you have to sit or lie down to recuperate. This symptom is present with other diseases as well, but with emphysema, the short-windedness is isolated—there aren't other signs of trouble to go with it. And it gets worse with time. Remember, the trouble here is in getting enough air out of your lungs—it's hard to exhale.

WHAT YOU CAN DO. If the tiny air sacs in your lungs are losing their ability to squeeze air out, it follows that anything you do to encourage this process will aid them. Recall ordinary breathing— I've discussed this previously. You inhale and exhale during the greater part of your life without really inhaling or exhaling as much as you can. If you were to *force* out and *force* in more air with each breath, you could move in and out considerably more total air. In emphysema, this is precisely what you've got to train yourself to do: Spend some time every day *forcing* in and *forcing* out all the air you can possibly squeeze with each breath. This means using your diaphragm and your abdominal muscles to their fullest capacity in breathing.

The next thing you can do is to practice forcing out air *against resistance* several times each day. The easiest way to do this is to take in as deep a breath as you can and then breathe out into a small closed container such as the end of your partially closed fist, a small tin can, or a dime store balloon. A plastic bag will do nicely. This exercise for your flabby air sacs is uncomfortable at first. Start slowly, perhaps with five or ten forced breaths into the balloon three times a day. Slowly increase the number until you're spending at least ten or fifteen minutes with these forced expirations three or four times a day.

You can restore reasonably good tone to your air sacs with this exercise. The exercise also helps to keep those sacs that haven't succumbed to the disease as yet in good tone. Of course, your regular exercise routines for the rest of your body help this cause because they make you breath harder and more deeply while you're doing them.

And you can stop smoking cigarettes altogether. Emphysema is one disease that won't permit the continuation of cigarettes. You can smoke a pipe, since most people don't inhale pipe smoke. You must be honest with yourself, however, and regard cigarettes as strictly prohibited from now on if you have emphysema.

If there is serious trouble with your lungs or if the process seems to be worsening, your doctor can prescribe medicines that help constrict air sacs artificially. These drugs can be quite helpful, and you should seek medical help for trouble you can't seem to handle.

If you're overweight, slim down promptly. The added burden of the increased oxygen supply necessary to support all that added weight only makes emphysema worse. Use what you've learned about mind control to start and keep up with those exhaling exercises constantly—perhaps just before your regular exercise routine. If the breathing exercises make you dizzy at first, don't be alarmed, just do them lying down until you're used to them. The dizziness will pass with a little time.

HOW TO DEAL WITH ASTHMA

Asthma is the clinical opposite of emphysema. Instead of it being difficult to get air out, you can't get enough oxygen *in* during asthma attacks.

Asthma is also a disease of lung air sacs. It occurs in sudden spasms as a rule, though some people with asthma wheeze most of the time. Emphysema, on the other hand, is a slowly progressive, chronic disease without sudden abrupt spasms. The air sacs during an asthmatic attack are clamped down like a collapsed balloon. Asthmatic people are air-hungry.

CAUSES. There are three main categories of asthma: Asthma caused from allergies, asthma caused from infections, and asthma caused by emotional turmoil. Many people have a mixture of two or even all three as the source of their trouble.

Asthma can be present in childhood. Emphysema always comes on in later years, no matter what the cause.

As a rule, childhood asthma presents itself during or following a heavy cold in the chest or on the heels of a bout of pneumonia, and it is ushered in by the sudden appearance of *wheezing*, the hallmark of an asthmatic attack. Even after the acute bout is gone, a doctor can listen to the chest of an asthmatic and tell that asthma is present—the wheezes persist between the spasms, but can't usually be heard without a stethoscope.

Any person with allergies to things that fly around in the air like pollens or dust or molds can become an asthmatic, but it doesn't follow that because you may have a good case of hay fever in the summer and fall of the year, you're going to have asthma. Some foods may trip an asthmatic attack. Most people with long-standing asthma notice that no matter what may have started their asthma, if they become upset from emotional problems, they have a typical asthma attack.

The nerves that control the muscles around the lung air sacs are branches of the very same ones that I discussed previously as controlling heart rate—the set of nerves that speeds up the heart also acts to relax the little air sacs. The set of nerves that slows your heart rate also acts to clamp down the air sacs. This explains why asthma can be emotionally caused. The cause of asthma when it's emotionally brought on is, of course, different from the cause when asthma is brought on by inhaling, say, air with heavy amounts of pollen in it. But the end result is the same. You can't tell one kind of asthma from another after it's started.

SYMPTOMS. Asthma always begins with spasms of wheezing. Wheezing is a noise that's produced by trying to force air in against the constricted air sacs. The loudest noises are during inhaling and the quietest noises are during exhaling. Both are loud enough to be heard across a room during an attack of asthma.

With the wheezing comes a feeling that you can't get enough air —that you may suffocate any minute if something isn't done. This suffocating feeling is enough to scare anyone, but you will get enough air.

An asthmatic may feel chest tightness during a chest cold, somewhat as though someone had your chest taped up so that breathing in is difficult. Exercising may produce this same feeling—like you'd just run a mile, but actually hadn't come close to such distance.

With asthma, the secretions in the air sacs, normally not enough to be noticed, increase. Since the air sacs are clamped down, the secretions that keep your lung linings moist can't get out; a choking sensation results, and coughing and phlegm is increased.

WHAT YOU CAN DO. (1) INFECTION TYPE. This type of asthma usually follows a chest infection, and may pop up with all infections in your chest from that time on. It may even come on with a sore throat or an infection far removed from your chest. Infection asthma doesn't occur too often. That is, since few people have continuous infections, their asthmatic attacks will be few and far between. I've discussed methods you can use in combating and preventing infection—good habits of blood sugar control. You need to follow these habits to the letter. If an infection does occur, the sooner it's terminated the sooner the asthma will disappear. If antibiotics are necessary, your doctor can prescribe them. For colds that aren't complicated with bacterial infection (colds are caused by viruses), the use of a drug that keeps your air sacs relaxed, free of thick secretions, and soothes their linings is in order. This medicine can be prescribed by your doctor and should be kept at hand all the time, even on vacations. It should be used at times and doses recommended by him, rather than all the time.

(2) ALLERGIC TYPE. The same applies here as with the infection type of asthma. The principles of blood sugar control apply. Allergies can be handled yet another way. Your doctor can desensitize you to most allergies after he tests you to find out what they all are. His advice on this should be followed, and if he recommends desensitizing you, you should be prepared to spend the year or two it takes to do an adequate job of this.

(3) EMOTIONAL TYPE. With this kind of asthma, you have an ideal situation in which you can put into practice what you've learned about mind control. Concentration on the problems you know bring on asthma will help you find ways to solve them. Concentration on the nerves that constrict the lung air sacs with suggestions that these nerves will calm down will help. Concentration on the air sacs themselves with suggestions that they relax is in order. I've witnessed asthma attacks disappear under hypnosis. This means that you can do the same thing using your own mind if you learn well the art of concentration. Asthma can be terminated after it starts, and it can be stopped before it starts if you have any warning at all that it's coming. Remember, concentrate on settling the nerves that cause your air sacs to constrict and on the air sacs themselves to relax. You can bring about excellent results in emotional asthma using your own mind.

HOW TO COPE WITH STOMACH ULCERS

Stomach ulcers are actually holes that are burned right into the inside lining of the stomach and upper intestinal tract. I say burned because that's just what the acid in your stomach does when the factors that ordinarily prevent it aren't working. The most common place for ulcers are really not in the stomach proper, but in the first part of the small intestine about two or three inches beyond the end of the stomach. This area is called the duodenum. About 90 per cent of "stomach ulcers" occur in the duodenum and about 10 per cent of them are in the stomach. The stomach is the place where food is digested into its simpler parts. Carbohydrate digestion starts in your mouth while you're chewing your food. This continues in the stomach. Proteins are split into smaller units in the stomach, then pass into your small intestine for final digestion. Fats are almost totally digested in the small intestine.

The stomach is much like the heart in that it is a hollow muscular bag under sensitive nerve and blood vessel control. That the nerves to your stomach begin to work hard just before meal time is demonstrated by the hunger pangs that start to plague you at this time. When stomach nerves begin this action, the glands that line the stomach begin to secrete their digestive juices. It's well to put something into your stomach at this time so this strongly acid juice won't have to digest the stomach lining itself!

CAUSES. The stomach is lined with several kinds of glands other than the ones that produce acid for digestion. Among these glands are those that produce the coating that protects the stomach lining from being digested by its own juices. Anything that disrupts the function of these coating glands will lay the lining bare to injury, and there are many things known to cause trouble to the protection glands.

The most common cause for an ulcer in the stomach or duodenum, as you may have guessed, is those pesky nerves again. Remember the nerves that slow the heart rate and constrict the air sacs in your lungs? These same nerves can stimulate the stomach glands to pour out large quantities of acid that really aren't needed in ordinary digestion. If this excess acid can penetrate the protection coating, you may have an ulcer.

These same nerves also stimulate the muscular walls of the stomach to churn and roll around. The "knot" that sometimes seems to be present right in your mid-section is caused by overactivity of this set of nerves.

Poor diet habits also cause a tremendous outpouring of digestive acid. Rich, spicy food eaten often and in entirely too much quantity over months or years can cause an ulcer. Being chronically ill from a number of diseases can cause the coating glands to become exhausted, with the stage then set for an ulcer.

SYMPTOMS. An ulcer starts with a gnawing pain in the mid-section of your abdomen. The pain is "deep," may have heartburn with it—a feeling of just having eaten a shaker full of pepper—and you may feel this "burn" all the way up your gullet. The pain from an ulcer is almost always relieved for a short time by eating food or drinking milk. But it comes right back again as soon as your stomach is empty. Nausea and vomiting are frequent in ulcer histories. Ulcer pain is usually high and in front of your abdomen, but if it travels, it may be felt in the back, of all places.

Less often, an ulcer forms so fast that there aren't many symptoms until complications have occurred. The two most frequent complications occur when the ulcer burns right through the wall of the stomach or small intestine and makes a hole, or when the ulcer burns through a small blood vessel in the intestine or stomach wall and bleeding occurs. Both these complications are surgical emergencies and require immediate attention in a hospital.

WHAT YOU CAN DO. Most ulcers can be prevented. A while ago, I said a common cause, the *most* common cause, of ulcers is overactivity of the large nerves that control the glands and the movement of the stomach walls. We have here a situation very similar to the lady in Chapter 7 who was prone to have spasms of rapid heart beat which she interpreted as heart attacks. People who get ulcers are people who can't let off that piled-up mental energy—that hostility or anger—and who take life's every frustration and setback to heart so thoroughly that their minds have to "bury" the incidents. Remember that when your mind has to "bury" these unpleasant parts of your life, you may be relieved of having to think much about them, but they are still a keg of dynamite. They have to be vented-off in some way. Besides the heart and lungs, the stomach is one of the mind's favorite sounding boards for unvented emotional energy. When all the pent-up steam from emotional problems comes boiling down the nerves to the stomach, you can literally feel your stomach recoil—it ties up in knots and you get heartburn! This doesn't necessarily mean you're going to have an ulcer. Everybody has had this experience at one time or another. But if it keeps up—if it continues to occur time and time again—something has to give, and it's the lining of your stomach or intestine that does, with an ulcer as the result.

How do you get rid of this buried nervous energy that can do so much damage over a period of time? *Blood sugar control!* Start those exercise routines. Get rid of the anger and frustration by taking it out on your muscles—they can't get ulcers!

Mind control is of the essence in preventing ulcers and in keeping yourself rid of them if you've already had one. You put your mind to work on the problems. What's making me tied up in knots? What's making me boiling mad, yet unable to ventilate it properly? Why am I a frustrated person? Ask your mind these questions. Sleep on them. Identify them one by one and *solve them!* Give your stomach a break. Don't make it take the brunt of your setbacks—your mind can help you resolve them, and the effort may save you an ulcer.

Diet to Follow

Diet habits at the first sign of indigestion are up for close review. Are you cutting down on the size of regular meals? Having snacks between meals? Drinking a generous portion of milk? Eliminating the rich, hard-to-digest foods from your diet? If the answer is no to any of these questions, you'd better review the chapter on diet. Notice how similar the rules of stomach care are to those of *good blood sugar control?* Almost identical! Antacids are the mainstay in medicating ulcers. Baking soda is not a good antacid to use with indigestion, even though it may be an effective antacid. Soda is absorbed into your system, and may cause trouble with the acid-alkali balance in your bloodstream, a delicate balance that must be maintained at all times. Select an antacid that's *not* absorbed into your system, but merely acts inside your stomach and intestine and that's all. Milk of magnesia is a good example of one such antacid. This compound is also a laxative, so you must be careful how much of it you use. Any antacid that says on the label that it contains magnesium trisilicate or magnesium carbonate is fine to use as an antacid. You can use such an antacid six to eight times a day if need be to get rid of heartburn and indigestion.

Your doctor may have to use more potent medicines to control ulcer symptoms. If the symptoms remain under good control, an ulcer will heal in two or three weeks without undue trouble. If you have grief with uncontrolled digestive disturbances, or if you see evidence of bleeding—vomiting of "coffee grounds" or black stools are signs of bleeding—see a medical expert for help.

DISEASES OF THE INTESTINES

The twelve to sixteen feet of small intestine that connect the stomach with the colon carries on the greater part of final digestion and absorbs the products into your system. Thanks to the digestive juices that come into the gut from the gall bladder and pancreas, the contents in the intestine are alkaline, just the opposite from the acid stomach contents. This is why there are rarely ever ulcers beyond the first few inches of small intestine. The rumbling and gurgling you hear and feel following meals is a sign that your small intestine is doing its job. When the food you eat is digested and there is nothing left but water, gas, and undigestible bulk, the contents are delivered into the large intestine, called the colon, where it's eliminated after most of the water has been reclaimed by the colon and absorbed back into your system.

The same nerves that control the stomach also control the small and large intestine. The gut is therefore subject to the same ills as the stomach, with the exception of ulcers. The one exception is ulcerative colitis, an unusual disease of the colon.

CAUSES. The most common affliction of the intestine is exactly the same as the stomach—the irritable gut, sometimes known as spastic enteritis or a spastic colon. Regardless of what name it's called, the cause is the same as that of its stomach counterpart—an overactive nervous system over which a lot of unresolved emotional problems are being channeled for lack of proper release before the mind "buries" them. As a consequence, your intestine falls ill to the symptoms produced by excess activity of its muscular walls, irritation of its inside lining from all the excess movement, and from failure to do its job of digesting and elimination properly.

SYMPTOMS. The irritable gut syndrome is characterized by one or more of the following symptoms:

1. Cramps after eating.
2. Gas, bloating and stuffed feeling. (Remember the stuffed-pig syndrome discussed in the second section?)
3. Either constipation or diarrhea, depending on what set of nerves is stimulated. (Either the set that slows down or the one that speeds up the intestinal activity respectively.)
4. The appearance of small amounts of blood and large amounts of mucous material in the stool.

WHAT YOU CAN DO. Much the same applies to the gut as applies to the stomach. Good principles of blood sugar control, including regular exercise, diet, and mind control, are the keys. Regarding diet, it can be said that anything to which you seem to be particularly sensitive should be cut down or eliminated. Beans, onions, fresh fruit, and the leafy vegetables are common offenders with an irritable gut. Any one of these foods can be eliminated entirely without harm. Regular vegetables easily compensate for the leafy ones. Any other leguminous vegetable (the ones that grow in pods) replaces beans. Onions are non-essential. There may be a few others. Fried and greasy foods, especially those that are heavily spiced, are rough on irritable colons. But these foods are also cut down as a regular part of blood sugar control, so you've already stopped one of the main categories that irritate your intestines.

Exercise serves a dual purpose. It restores tone to the muscular abdominal wall, therefore also the intestine, and it serves as an excellent outlet for excess nervous energy.

Mind control can stop cramps. Concentrating on relaxation of your intestinal muscles can stop or drastically reduce cramps. Concentrating on intestinal muscle activity can help to step up a sluggish, constipated colon. If you happen to be a person who is troubled with an irritable gut of any kind, you'll find that heavy smoking and drinking has a particularly bad effect on the condition. Cigarettes and alcohol should be curtailed 75 per cent with any disease of the intestinal tract, whether it starts in the mouth, in the rectum, or anywhere between.

DISEASES OF THE GALL BLADDER

The gall bladder has plagued mankind for centuries. It's a small muscular bag, just under the right part of the liver, that stores bile as it is manufactured by the liver. During intestinal digestion, it contracts, emptying "gall" (bile) into the intestinal tract to aid in protein and fat digestion. This little carrying case for bile can really cause trouble. The gall bladder gets into trouble most often with women who are in their middle years and overweight. The reason for it is that its inside lining becomes irritated and inflamed with the constant barrage of excess fats in the diet. Infection may be the result of such chronic irritation and that's when an acute attack occurs during which there is fever, chills, and a severe pain in the right upper abdomen that may radiate around the waist to the right shoulder blade. This kind of pain is typical of gall bladder irritation from any cause.

CAUSES. Poor attention to blood sugar control again! For every person of normal weight who has gall bladder difficulties, there are fifty that are overweight. This includes infections (sometimes called bilious attacks or gall bladder colic, gall stones, and just overactivity of this organ. People with gall bladder trouble are generally out of condition. That is, they're soft and flabby. They are slow, sloth-like people to whom activity in the physical sense is practically unheard of. They also drink too much alcohol.

The cause of gall stone formation is still not definite as yet, but this much is certain: If there is the "soft life," the lazy sluggish attitude about life in general, and poor judgment regarding diet, there can be gall stones and they can really cause trouble.

SYMPTOMS. A gall bladder attack of most any kind is generally ushered in about an hour or two following an especially rich and fatty meal. It begins with bloating and fullness in the upper abdomen and progresses to pain that may be constant but with definite "waves" or spasms of much worse pain in the upper abdomen and back. If infection is present, fever and chills may then start. Nausea and vomiting are the rule with any severe attack. A person having a gall bladder attack may throw up "black bile" which means that the intestine has gone into spasm at the point where the bile canal empties into it, and the bile has nowhere to go but in reverse. It flows into the stomach and is upchucked.

The course of gall stone disease may occur over several months or years. But the attacks generally follow the same characteristic pattern: Food, one or two hours delay, gas and bloating, then waves of pain in the right upper side of the abdomen.

WHAT YOU CAN DO. Get over those lazy ways! Get active. Peal off those excess flabby pounds. Manage your diet as you've learned in blood sugar control. Once you have gall bladder trouble, the same rules apply, only more stringently. Cut drinking and smoking to the bare line, and eliminate both entirely if you can. Acute trouble with the gall bladder demands that you have medical help—seek it out if you're at all suspicious.

Once gall stones have formed and are discovered on X-ray, they'd best be taken out surgically. Following recovery, the rules of blood sugar control apply strictly. If gall stones are present and aren't removed surgically, they almost always cause trouble of a kind you can't afford. They (stones) may erode through the gall bladder wall and get into your abdominal cavity where they may raise all kinds of havoc. They may pass into the canal that carried bile to the intestine where they may block off the flow of this digestive juice. When this happens, gall bladder jaundice is the result—the bile can't get into the intestine, so it backs up into the liver, then into the bloodstream, where it causes your skin to turn yellow and itch intensely. None of these conditions are compatible with continued good health, so if you have gall stones, have them removed and start the basics of good blood sugar control immediately thereafter!

DISEASES OF THE KIDNEY

The most common disease in the kidney is infection or a kidney stone. They occur together very frequently. Anyone with repeated kidney infections is suspect of kidney stone, and a search for stones should be launched. Anything that causes obstruction in the urinary tract from the outlet of the bladder to the kidney itself can start an infection. This happens because anything that blocks the flow of urine out of the kidney causes urine to stagnate, and the germs normally present in the urine (remember urine is a *waste* product) are allowed to multiply causing infection.

CAUSES. Since obstruction anywhere along the urinary tract can cause infection, it follows that a narrowing of the urinary channel anywhere along the tract can cause trouble. The urinary tract is considered to be from the edge of each kidney, where the tubes that convey urine to the bladder start, to the outside where urine is discharged.

In a man, prostate trouble is a common cause of urinary problems because this gland surrounds the outlet from the bladder. If the prostate swells up for any number of reasons, it can block off flow of urine from the bladder. If the ring of muscle around the neck of the bladder (the lower end of the bladder where urine is conveyed to the outside during urination) is irritated or doesn't function properly, the urine is blocked off from getting to the outside. If there is a urinary stone in either of the two tubes that lead from the kidney to the bladder, urine is prevented from reaching the bladder, and infection starts as a result.

SYMPTOMS. Urinary infection begins with trouble in the act of urination. It may start with an urgency and frequency of urination far in excess of usual. Together with urgency and frequency, there is burning when the urine is being passed or just after the bladder is emptied. These signs mean infection and must be dealt with medically.

If the infection is in the bladder or higher up in either kidney, fever and chills may be present. And pain may be present along the area of the tube leading from the kidney to the bladder—in the flank—in the groin or in the lower part of the abdomen. This pain, somewhat like that of the gall bladder, is usually crampy—colicky —it occurs in waves. The pain with a kidney stone is exactly the same, only more intense. It doubles you over when the wave of pain starts.

WHAT YOU CAN DO. The prevention of kidney infection and stones is the same. Remember that your kidneys depend absolutely on a constant ample supply of water to do their job. Remember also that it's no strain to your kidneys to have to concentrate urine (make it stronger), but when your kidneys are forced to do this often and over long periods of time, the excess concentration and reduced amount of urine may be enough to start an infection along the urinary tract. So the way to treat and to prevent kidney infection and stones is to insure a constant intake of an adequate amount of fluids every day. This is particularly true during long periods of hot weather when you lose more water by sweating. It means you must drink the equivalent of 10 or 12 large full glasses of water every day at minimum. More during hot weather.

The basics of blood sugar control demand routine exercise. This, in itself, demands more fluids than usual—give in to the urge to drink fluids of any kind after exercising. Alcohol is *not* considered a fluid because it diminishes water in your system. Alcohol consumption demands even more water than usual—if you drink alcohol even moderately, you need up to three times the normal amounts of water every day!

Exercise also speeds up the blood flow through your kidneys. Waste is eliminated more efficiently, and more urine is formed.

Both kidney stones and infections demand medical attention. Seek it out if you suspect either, then get with the blood sugar control!

DISEASES OF THE JOINTS

Rheumatism and arthritis are two of the scourges of the human race. They've been with us longer and have been described by the ancients longer than perhaps any other disease. Anyone who has ever been or is afflicted with arthritis is easy prey to a host of charlatans and quacks who at least understand one important thing about arthritis: No matter with what the disease is treated, it will eventually improve—even disappear for a time—only to recur again later. It follows that if you happen to be taking alfalfa concentrate (a commonly used treatment by the quacks), you will naturally praise alfalfa as "a great cure" when your arthritis gets better or disappears for a time. You could have produced exactly the same "cure" by using rhubarb and honey, anise oil and caraway seeds, by bathing in "radium pools," or even by using cortisone. The point is, there is really no permanent *cure* for arthritis —only relief and proper living of life compatible with the particular case. In your car, when the universal joint gives out, it has to be replaced. Proper lubrication before this time may prolong its life, but once it gives out, there is no getting around its replacement. Your joints are the same. Once they give out, transplants have so far not succeeded in replacing the human joint. They may some-day, then arthritis will be "cured" in the full sense of the word. But until transplants are successful with joints, we must content ourselves with the prevention of this malady called rheumatism, arthritis, lumbago, or whatever.

CAUSES. A variety of things cause arthritis. I've discussed with you the hereditary parts of certain diseases like diabetes. The same applies to arthritis—there is definitely a hereditary factor in some cases of arthritis. The hereditary factor may be present, yet arthritis may not appear. Why is this? Just like other hereditary diseases, there must be an environmental (local) factor that, together with the hereditary part of the disease, makes joints stiff, painful, and sometimes useless.

Trauma is another cause of arthritis, and it's becoming more prevalent. Trauma, or injury to a joint, can induce arthritis whether or not there are either hereditary or local factors present. A football player is clipped—injures his knee—is laid up for the season. He may play on the injured leg another season, with the firm conviction that his leg has healed from the twisting and tearing the ligaments in his knee joint sustained. But he will have arthritis in this knee a couple of years later.

A carpenter slips off a roof and lands on his tail bone. He sustains a compression injury to his lower spine. This heals up and he's able to return to work some time later without apparent trouble. Five years later, he begins to have lumbago in his spine—another way of saying arthritis in the injured joints in his spinal column.

And there is our old friend, infection. A steel worker gets clipped with a sharp edge on an I-beam, it hits his hip. An infection starts and involves his hip joint. Two years later, he begins to have arthritis in this previously infected joint.

SYMPTOMS. Arthritis causes pain and stiffness in or around joints. The pain and stiffness don't have to be right in the joint, they can be in the ligaments and tendons around the joint and also in the muscles.

In some kinds of arthritis, there is swelling in the joint. Rheumatoid arthritis is a "sweller." In other forms of arthritis the skin around the joint gets red and warm to the touch. Gout is such a type. When the acute phase of the arthritis is over, the pain, stiffness, redness, and swelling slowly disappear. Sometimes altogether; sometimes leaving a trace of stiffness and pain, but not as severe as previously.

WHAT YOU CAN DO. You can keep those joints and ligaments and tendons and muscles limbered up. You can avoid putting yourself in positions of recurring injury. If you have an injured joint, you can do all you can to get it back to proper function again, and you can stop whatever it was you were doing so it won't happen again. You can take care of the small infections around joints so they don't get to be big ones. And you can exert good blood sugar control, more than usual, if your family tree has arthritis in it.

Any time you have an acute arthritis that has swelling and warmth in and around the joints involved, regardless of how it started, you need medical advice. Get it immediately and follow the principles of sugar control!

SURGERY, AND HOW TO RECOVER FROM IT

Did you ever stop to think how tough a patient makes it on a surgeon when, during an abdominal operation, the surgeon has to cut through six inches of pure flab before he even reaches the muscle layer? Did you ever consider how tough you make things on yourself when you allow your muscles to get soft and flabby, and then wonder why you aren't doing too well after an operation? Why it takes you three weeks to be able to walk comfortably instead of five days or a week? There is only one answer to such questions. You simply haven't taken care of that blood sugar as you should. Surgery in this day and age is a far cry from what it was twenty years ago, but there are still far too many post-operative complications. Most of these complications could be avoided with a little attention to the principles of blood sugar control.

FEAR. The fear of surgery still looms large in anyone's mind. The fear is natural enough, but entirely unfounded and unrealistic. If technique has permitted the removal of such a vital organ as a heart and its replacement by another, why should anyone fear a relatively uncomplicated bit of surgery as an exploratory procedure of the abdomen or removal of a gall bladder? Armed with the forces at your command, gained from Chapter 5 on the mind and its control, you can prepare yourself to be calm, relaxed, cooperative, and actually eager for the procedure so that you can be healthy and robust again following whatever surgery you may need.

Fear is always the dread of the unknown or the unexpected. Ask your surgeon to go over what's going to happen—how he's going to do the operation. You'll be amazed at how simple it is. You'll also get rid of that unknown quantity, a good riddance and the way to eliminate fear. And you can rest assured that modern anesthesiology will be more than up to the task of making it possible for you to be quite asleep and having peaceful dreams right in your room before you're wheeled to surgery. You'll never know it happened!

PAIN. It's been proven beyond a shadow of a doubt that pain following surgery is a product of fear and regression—a going back to a child-like state of mind that dictates complete rejection of anything that's uncomfortable. This means that most pain is the result of poor habits of mind control. Remember those patients in Chapter 5 that were able to overcome pain. If they can do it, so can you.

COMPLICATIONS. Most after-surgery complications can be traced to poor conditioning. Consider blood clots, the nemesis of surgery a generation ago. The only reason this complication has been practically eliminated is that people are required to get up out of bed and start using their muscles the very day of the operation rather than being allowed to lie on their backsides for days without moving. The blood in the veins of the legs depends absolutely on the action of the leg muscles to move it upward and back into the circulation again. No muscle action in the legs: No return of blood to the circulation. This spells *clot.*

Chest complications lead the list of after-surgery troubles. The reason? Lack of proper breathing and lack of activity. Deep breathing—15 forced deep breaths every hour during the day—

may mean the difference between rapid recovery and a two week longer stay in the hospital with a lung infection or a blood clot.

HEALING. The healing of any wound, especially a surgical one, depends on the promotion of an active circulation of blood in and around the wound. How is this done? By early ambulation and physical activity. It doesn't stand up any more that a patient must be quiet and not "strain his incision." He must be active and must make those muscles around the wound contract. If he doesn't, healing just won't be efficient. The better tone those muscles have been accustomed to, the better and more efficient will be healing. And it's been shown that even a *little* movement around the site of a fracture makes the fracture heal faster and more solidly! And what do the healing powers of your body need to do their job? They need adequate protein, carbohydrate, and fat—in other words, they need good basic attention to blood sugar control before and after surgery.

SUMMARY

1. Emphysema and asthma can be prevented and controlled by good habits of blood sugar control. If either one enters the picture, *blood sugar control* principles apply in their management.
2. The most common affliction of the stomach and intestinal tract has to do with improper channeling of emotional energy over the large nerves that control these organs. Mind control and proper attention to diet can prevent and cure most of these ills, including indigestion, bloating, cramps, the irritable gut syndrome, and bowel dysfunction. Bring to bear what you've learned about blood sugar control.
3. Gall stones and kidney stones and infections in both these organs are caused by obstruction along their drainage tracts. These can be prevented by proper diet, proper intake of fluids, and exercise.
4. Diseases of the joints, ligaments, and muscles can be traced to poor conditioning, trauma (injury), infection, and heredity. You can control everything but heredity in preventing crippling disease.

5. Surgery requires a patient's preparation. Ask your surgeon questions to overcome fear, and practice mind control principles to get yourself back into the realm of the healthy again following surgery. Good principles of blood sugar control apply the second you wake up from the anesthesia.

10

How to Add Healthful Years to Your Life and Reverse the Rigors of Aging

As long as men have been mortal, they've approached the aging process with a certain amount of dread, a certain amount of regret, and with little dignity and grace. I want to talk about aging and the aging process in this section. I will talk not only about what aging means to your body, but also in relation to your mind. The so-called secrets of spry longevity will be covered, as well as how you can plan your golden years to the best advantage.

I want to talk about retirement and what it means to you and your blood sugar, how you may avoid retirement rot, and what you can do to head off senility (infirmity of mind).

The blood sugar picture after age 60 years will be covered, and how you can maintain all the principles of blood sugar control in spite of the slower pace of later years; why blood sugar control is important during this time of later life.

THE AGING PROCESS

There are many definitions for aging. The closest to home is the one that put it thus: Aging occurs when a person stops spinning his wheels and traveling in circles and starts walking in straight lines. The exact time in life that those "clinkers" I've discussed with you start to accumulate in cells and start aging them varies a good deal from person to person. I've found, though, that people who seem to retain their youthful appearance beyond the usual time, seem to lose it rapidly once the process starts, so it doesn't follow that the man of forty who looks and acts twenty-five or thirty will outlast anyone else who seems to age at a more normal rate.

Aging starts in different cells at different times. Endurance and stamina seem to be first affected—these two qualities are grounded in muscles, nerves, and the will. Of these three sites—muscles, nervous tissue, and the mind—it's nervous tissue that usually stands up against aging the poorest. Nerve cells, whether they're in the long nerve trunk that runs from the spinal cord to the foot (the sciatic nerve) or whether they're in the part of the brain that makes up the area that controls your heart beat, are vulnerable to aging. One reason nerve cells are the first to age is that they require more oxygen, more nutrition, and more elimination of waste products than other less highly specialized cells. Nerve cells metabolize at a much faster rate than, say, skin cells. Not only does it turn over energy at a much faster rate, but nervous tissue is subject to more constant internal change than other cells. Even at rest, nerve cells must rejuvenate while being constantly bombarded by a host of impulses from the brain and spinal cord—the switchboard never stops its functions.

There are several influences that start aging in any cell. The first hint of aging appears to come at that point in development when all cells in the body cease to increase their total numbers —when they no longer have the ability to divide and form *new* cells. For most humans, this point is reached between the ages of 18 and 21 years—the period of final growth. This has nothing to do with the *size,* say, of your biceps muscle—this muscle and all others can be developed to get bigger, but no new cells are added with this enlargement. The ones that are already there simply get bulkier.

But what of the skin? Isn't this an exception? The outside layer of skin cells, including the ones that make your hair, do indeed replenish themselves, but these cells are just a coating, so to speak, and they're made from the base layer of your skin—the red layer that's exposed when you have an injury that scrapes. These skin cells at the base don't multiply—their number remains quite constant. The pink or black or brown outer covering of your skin isn't the *living* cells of skin—they're merely the products of the living layer.

The tiny power plant in each of the trillions of cells in your body is called the nucleus. The nucleus contains an exact duplicate of the original set of genes and chromosomes that started out in the single cell you once were when your parents' sperm and ovum united to form the unique individual that made you. There are literally thousands of scientists throughout the world today who make it their life work to study the single living human cell. Each year, they unlock dozens of the secrets contained within its fantastically complicated mechanism. Exactly what slows down the machinery inside the cell and causes the "clinkers" to pile up, to retard, the cell's function (the cellular basis for what we call aging) will probably be completely understood physically and chemically in the not too distant future. When this becomes known, the means to arrest—perhaps even halt—the aging process will be at hand.

BLOOD SUGAR CONTROL

Thus far in this book, everything I've discussed with you has had as its basis the maintenance of such a state of metabolism in the cells of your body that their peak efficiency of performance is attained and kept that way. It's just this problem of aging for which your blood sugar control now sets the stage. Not only will you feel well and enjoy good health with adequate blood sugar control, but you'll also age gracefully and easily. Consider these principles briefly again:

DIET. I've yet to see a really unhealthy person over the age of 60 who kept his diet under control and managed to stay slim. This isn't to say nothing serious ever happens to a slender person. What I'm saying is that diet control is the more important the more advanced your age. *Remember those arteries!* The ones that supply blood and oxygen and sugar to the cells of your brain and heart. The hardening process progresses at a rapid rate after fifty *if you don't keep the fats and excess carbohydrates down.* Your metabolism slows with aging. Your cells don't require the tremendous energy turnover they once did. What it took at twenty years to keep you going is now too much. So watch the height-weight-frame tables earlier in this book closely and keep that weight in line!

Women past fifty have a tougher time with this problem than men. The reason is tied up with menopause. After menopause, or after surgery that removes the uterus and ovaries, women put weight on more easily. The reason is that the endocrine feedback pathway that existed between ovaries and pituitary (the master endocrine gland) is broken when the ovaries cease to produce their normal amounts of estrogen. For a while, the pituitary continues to try to stimulate the ovaries just as it did each month before menopause. This stimulation also increases the appetite and causes the tissues to retain fluid, again, just as before a monthly period in the premenopausal days. The net result is that weight goes up!

Eliminating excess salt from your diet, as well as being extra careful with your intake of calories, will block this tendency to gain weight if you're in the period of menopause.

MUSCLE TONE. Take a good look at people over fifty. Note how the majority have let their muscles get very soft and flabby. This, together with lack of attention to their weight, has had the effect of increasing their age!

If you've started your muscle toning routines, and if you've made them a regular part of your life, you'll automatically have insured yourself a long life of comfort and productivity. If you've reached the fifties or sixties and haven't gotten around to this vital blood sugar measure to halt the aging process, *start your routines now*—there's still time to do worlds of good. In a short time you'll feel so much better that you won't want to quit. In fact, you'll feel uncomfortable if you skip a day or two!

When you start your exercise routine late in life, remember that you're not trying to do what a twenty-year-old does. You don't need this much anyway, because you'll find that your muscle tone and vigor respond without the exertion that a twenty-year-old must go through to achieve the same results. Start with the simple things—walking, jogging within limits set by your lungs, and isometric-type routines. As you slowly work up the *time* spent with exercise and your endurance increases, you can progress to a few calisthenics—again, within the limits set by your lungs and heart.

Riding a bicycle and swimming are excellent general toning-up activities, but stop and rest when you feel fatigue. Do your routine regularly and increase your endurance slowly. If you have a physical condition that requires treatment, consult with your medical expert to see what he sets as limits to your exercising.

MIND CONTROL. What I've said previously about your mind and aging bears repeating. There is no more important step you can take than to keep your mind active, alert and challenged at every turn. If you've not reached the age of fifty or more, the first thing to be done is a critical appraisal of your interests and hobbies—your pastimes and your leisure-time activities. The great American tragedy, in my opinion, is the pasturing out at retirement of people sixty or sixty-five years old who are ill-prepared, ill-suited, and even ill-inclined to continue a good life without "the old grind" they've become accustomed to. Furthermore, even folks who are self-employed, like farmers and business owners, I find have not prepared themselves properly for the golden years of retirement.

The time to start this preparation isn't on the spur of the moment, when you're going to retire next week. The time is *now*. A careful evaluation of your interests, your likes and dislikes, your tinkering urges—all these must be brought to bear in this planning. What about all those things you thought you'd always like to do, but never got around to it? What about all those frustrated urges to create? To make? To mold or to paint? You can build a whole new life around any one or several of such urges never before realized.

Reading, one of the most cherished pastimes of many people, isn't much thought of today as an activity with which to further the mind's potential. But there's nothing like it. Haven't you ever been puzzled by questions, such as the way your own government works? From the county level right up to the federal government? Take this opportunity to find out. Become an informed citizen while you're at it.

THE KEYS TO LIFE AFTER SIXTY

REGULARITY. Being well regulated is different from getting into a rut. Being regular with your habits of blood sugar control is just the opposite; in fact, it means keeping yourself *from* getting into ruts!

To put aside *time* for doing things is not getting into a rut. It's the leavening influence that putting aside time brings. It's this regularity that's desirable as opposed to the whims of meaningless starts and stops in your life. It's a regularity of challenge, a regularity of health and wisdom. And it's a regularity of body machinery that performs much better when it's taken care of on a regular basis than when it's neglected.

Regularity deals with body, mind, and activity. It deals with keeping your muscles, nerves, and endocrine glands subject to excellent working order—exercise routines, diet control, and conditioning. Your body at sixty years can't and won't respond and keep responding day in and day out to stresses and strains as it did at twenty. Although you may find yourself requiring actually less sleep for rejuvenation, periods of complete relaxation on a regular basis are indicated.

Regular meals with well-regulated amounts of protein, carbohydrate, and fat, and the between meal snacks you've already learned about are important to you at this stage of life. Your biological clock, the mechanism that regulates digestion, endocrine gland activity, and metabolism, among others, works better and more efficiently if you're on regular schedule.

ACTIVITY. The question of youth versus senility can be summarized in one word: *Mind.* People who haven't taken the time to develop good habits of mind become senile. The word senile in this sense refers to the "crotchety old man or the nice little old lady" who can't manage by himself, who must be dressed, fed, and guided from trouble throughout most of every day. Senile people are the ones that get to be "hard to handle" in that they're unable to keep themselves clean and can't get along with anyone—they're the irrascible and argumentative ones! Everything they do and every word they say is critical of their surroundings and the people in it. Often, such cranks have to be "put away" for their own protection. I'm certain you've seen many of these folks; you may have someone like this in your own family. Take a good look at these pitiable older people. Is this the way you want to be remembered? Is this how you want your golden years to culminate? Of course it isn't.

If you observe older people carefully, you'll notice the signs: generalized weakness of muscles and joints; a tendency to remember only those events that occurred in their lives in the far distant past; constant repetition of the same words or subject over and over again; confusion as to where they are or have been; disorientation in place and time; inability to concentrate or follow thoughts, and so on. Behind this irreversible picture lies the old spectre of hardened arteries, which lead to lowered function of mind and body, which leads to—senility. We've talked about the facts that bear on hardening of those important arteries in the brain. You've learned how to prevent artery hardening through good habits of blood sugar maintenance: Diet, exercise, and mind control. You can now directly observe the *results of neglecting blood sugar control* by looking at senility. You can prevent this senile picture from settling in if you're willing to do what's necessary to keep your mind and body from deteriorating. It's never too late to start. If you can notice the signs, you can still head them off!

Whatever your leaning, whatever your ambition after retirement, *keep active at it.*

If you must be hospitalized, preparation before you go home can spell the difference between a reasonably good return to normality or the start of decay following conditions that put you in there in the first place. I can think of any number of patients who have sustained heart attacks or strokes who probably would be glued to their beds at home today were it not for the fact that it was shown to them before they ever left the hospital that they could, indeed, do many things they didn't think possible. People find with strokes, for example, that not *all* muscles are paralyzed on the side involved. Once they learn how to put strength back into these remaining muscles and to use the muscles they more or less once ignored on the side that isn't affected, they immediately have their self-confidence restored. Some people seem to fear that their minds have been ruined by such attacks. Your mind is perfectly capable of adapting itself even to a severe stroke—your mind's recovery will be the rule, depending on how well you've mastered the art of developing it beforehand.

LIFTING YOUR SPIRITS

If you've never had occasion to come to terms with the business of spirit, the years after fifty afford an excellent opportunity.

Coming to terms with spirit means bringing yourself into harmony with the world around you as you see both in your mind. Your spirit is that uniquely human quality you share with 3.5 billions of people in this world. Your spirit is what makes you human and what unites you with other humans.

How unfortunate it is that many hundreds of thousands of individuals are born, live out their lives, and die without every moving into harmony with either themselves or with the outside world of human beings! I suppose that a busy life active with the job of family rearing and breadwinning is a reasonable excuse with most people. There is a point in life where, for final justification of all that has gone before, you need to step back from the mainstream and carefully observe what you see. Observe and evaluate the course and direction of your life as well as those of your fellow humans. You may well question whether what you see is the way it should be. Or whether anything can be done about it. Or where you've fitted in all this time, and what changes will take place during your later years that may shift your position. This is good. This will bring you in contact with your spirit and lift it to still higher levels of aspiration and achievement. Failing in this "grand perspective," your spirit may wither away and finally become dormant. And this alternative will spell a deep rut indeed —one out of which you may find it impossible to climb.

Some people find the meaning of spirit in their religions. I think this is an excellent place to look. Others find it in broadening their education—through reading, through doing, and through innovating (finding new approaches to problems). Whatever way you choose, rest assured that it can't help but further the cause for your spirit, no matter what you may think about the place of spirit in your life at the present time.

I've seen a good many examples of this "moving of spirit," but one of the most interesting, I think, was a man whom I met following his retirement as the chief sales executive for an international oil company. He had been the perfect example of the "big wheel." He jetted across oceans to close deals; he had unlimited expense accounts; he was the typical big smile and hand-shake artist whose life was spent spreading what he thought was his company's good image at home and abroad.

Toward the end of his active career, he began to have misgivings—doubts about both his company, its so-called image, and about what it was he was actually doing all this time with his worldly hopping about. When this man finally did retire at sixty-five, he looped into a depressive stage and developed all kinds of aches, pains, and symptoms, even though he enjoyed almost perfect health. A little probing brought up all kinds of doubts about the importance of his job, about the hypocrisy of modern business practices, and about his own role as a human being all these years. The man was not a senile, sentimental old fool wishing to regain his youth. He was a well-educated, well-rounded, interested individual who hadn't bothered before to ask himself the question, "Why?" Why am I telling people one thing and doing another? Why does the company image need glossing if it's so good anyway? Why do I spend so much time buttering up important people when they really aren't so important except as business for the company? All these and other questions seriously concerned this man.

To answer some of his more difficult questions, the man took to the subject of philosophy (remember, I've discussed philosophy in Chapter 5). He wanted to get to the basic issues of this thing called life and all its problems. He chose a good subject. He became so engrossed in it, as a matter of fact, that he decided to enroll in evening classes in philosophy at a local university. He became so proficient in his subject that he is now consulting expert and guest lecturer in the philosophy of business at this university!

There is no limit to what heights your spirit can move you, as this man's experience shows. If you've learned the principles of blood sugar control, moving your spirit should prove no task, and it will come as a natural sequence of attention to diet, exercise, and mind control.

THE MOST IMPORTANT CONTRIBUTION YOU'LL EVER MAKE

The process of aging brings you to the most important crossroad in your life. At last, you are in the position of bringing to those around you and to your community the most precious gift a man or woman can bestow: Wisdom.

It's perhaps unfortunate, but a fact of life, that intelligence and new knowledge does not carry its own wisdom with it. Wisdom comes only with the broadest experience in the myriad situations that make up a lifetime. This canon, or rule, or equation, or whatever you may wish to call it, is not easily learned. Youth doesn't believe it, as a matter of fact, and it's up to you at this point to get across to young people the idea that wisdom is a gift of virtue, and you're in an unbelievably good position to add this measure of life's wisdom to the sum total of their knowledge.

The calm rational influence on younger people is quite underplayed today. Youth has been raised to believe that its ideas are the final and ultimate answer to the world's problems. To a degree, young people have a right to feel this way, but they've carried it to the extreme. They need the guidance of wisdom whether they realize it or not.

Today's youngsters are unsettled chiefly because they're impatient, confused (and rightfully so), and frightened. It's time you older people took a hand in straightening the situation out for them. It's time they learned how to put starch in their backbone, straighten up, and grasp the world as it is, not as some people would like to paint it for them. And it's time they were given the opportunity to develop guts—fortitude—courage, or whatever the best term may be. These attributes aren't something young people are born with. They have to be learned. You're the ones to teach youth!

SUMMARY

1. The problems concerned with aging are chiefly the result of inattention to the basic habits of *blood sugar control*. If you've neglected these principles, it isn't too late to start *now*.
2. Regularity is different from being in a rut. Regularity in life after sixty years is a must—regularity of diet, exercise, and mind control. Senility is the result of neglecting your mind. You can avoid senility by keeping your mind active in dozens of different ways. The key is to *face challenges—to make* your mind stay active.

Supplemental Aids for Your Blood Sugar Control Program

A. REDUCING DIETS

STRICT

BREAKFAST. One slice of bread—toasted or plain.
One egg—poached or boiled.
One cup (8 ounces) skim milk.
One small orange or ½ cup (4 ounces) orange juice.

LUNCH. Three soda crackers.
Two cold-cut slices or ½ cup cottage cheese.
Four ounces (½ cup) skim milk.
Two tablespoons raisins or one small apple.

DINNER. Any amount of *uncooked* asparagus, broccoli, brussels sprouts or tomatoes.
One serving of beets, carrots, peas, turnips or squash (one serving equals 4 ounces or ½ cup).
Two slices of any meat *or* ½ cup (4 ounces) fish *or* two tablespoons peanut butter on crackers.
Four ounces of skim milk.
Four ounces pineapple *or* two of any dried fruit *or* ½ small banana.

LESS STRICT.

BREAKFAST.   ½ cup (4 ounces) cooked cereal of any kind, *or* 6 ounces ¾ cup) of dry cereal with skim milk.
One egg—poached or boiled.
One cup skim milk.
½ cup any berries, *or* ½ cup any fruit juice.
One teaspoon margarine (one square).

LUNCH.   Two slices of bread, *or* ½ cup cooked noodles or spaghetti.
Two frankfurters, *or* two slices cheddar cheese.
½ cup skim milk.
Two cups any berries, *or* one peach *or* one apple, *or* two of any dried fruit.
One tablespoon cream, *or* one teaspoon mayonnaise.

DINNER.   Any amount of *uncooked* cabbage, cauliflower, eggplant, greens, or squash.
One serving of onions, turnips, or carrots.
½ cup cooked rice, *or* two slices of bread, *or* one baked potato.
Three slices of any meat or cheese, *or* ¾ cup of any fish.
½ cup skim milk.
¼ of any melon, *or* a dozen grapes, *or* two any dried fruit.
Two tablespoons salad dressing, *or* two teaspoons cooking fat, *or* two squares margarine.

At any meal or at any time between meals, the following foods may be taken in any quantity since they have negligible calories:

COFFEE	LEMON
TEA	UNSWEETENED GELATIN
CLEAR BROTH	RENNET TABLETS
BOUILLON (FAT-FREE)	UNSWEETENED CRANBERRIES
DRY MUSTARD	UNSWEETENED PICKLES
ANY SUGAR SUBSTITUTE	SPICES
VINEGAR	SEASONINGS
LOW CALORIE SOFT DRINKS	

In addition, the following vegetables may be used at any meal or between meals so long as they are eaten uncooked:

ASPARAGUS	EGGPLANT	MUSTARD	ROMAINE
BROCCOLI	ESCAROLE	STRING BEANS	RADISHES
BRUSSELS SPROUTS	GREENS	SPINACH	WATERCRESS
CABBAGE	PARSLEY	TURNIP GREENS	TOMATOES
POKE	CHARD	LETTUCE	RHUBARB
SAUERKRAUT	COLLARDS	MUSHROOMS	PEPPERS
CHICORY	DANDELION	OKRA	CELERY
CUCUMBER	KALE	SUMMER SQUASH	

As you continue to diet, you'll learn how to substitute. For example, if you don't eat fruit for breakfast, you can substitute one strip of bacon from which the grease has been drained. If you don't eat bread or toast, crackers can be substituted. If you'd rather have all bread or toast, cereal can be eliminated. But no cheating! In general, meats should be baked, broiled, or boiled. Don't fry them in oil or fats. If you do use oil or fats for preparing meats, eliminate both bread and margarine from the allowable foods that meal.

When preparing vegetables from the cooked list, don't add flour or extra fat to them. It isn't necessary to use special foods. If you like canned fruit, buy it water-packed rather than packed in syrup.

Remember, it isn't wise to skip meals. Remember, too, that alcoholic drinks are heavy in carbohydrates—if you drink them while dieting, you must cut the amount of food at the next meal roughly in half to balance out!

Once you have your weight in hand, you may gradually slip away from your diet depending on your exercise routine. As long as your weight remains steady, you're getting enough to eat. If you have your weight steadied, begin your exercise routine, and find you're losing weight again, you need more food—don't hesitate to eat it!

B. ALTERNATE EXERCISES FOR VARIOUS MUSCLE GROUPS

I. FACE

Your forehead muscles are controlled by the same ones that elevate your eyebrows. Practice in front of a mirror elevating both eyebrows to their fullest height, then pull them down into a deep "scowl" position. Repeat this maneuver several times. Later, practice elevating both brows, then lowering just your left brow, then just the right.

When you can control either side at will, your frontal muscles will be in good shape, and many of those wrinkles will be ironed out.

The muscles around your eyes are important because they are the "bags" beneath your eyes when they're out of condition. These muscles also get the dark circles in them and cause you to appear ill. Exercise these muscles by pulling your eyes into a squint. This is done by pulling up your cheeks toward your eyes and smiling broadly at the same time. With this forced "squint" held firmly in place, close both eyelids forcibly until you feel the muscles that encircle them pull tightly, then relax. Repeat this several dozen times.

The muscles that move your eye balls around can be exercised by simply moving your eyes rapidly in all conceivable directions until your vision is blurred from the rapid movement.

The muscles that exercise your mouth are used simply by pulling your mouth into a forced smile and holding it for a few seconds. This can be alternated with an enforced droop of the mouth which also pulls your chin muscles inwardly. Alternately pursing your lips into a tight round puckered shape, then into lips-turned outwardly, then lips pulled to the sides, will exercise the muscles that surround your mouth. Forcibly opening your mouth, utilizing the muscles beneath your chin, and holding this position will aid in getting rid of the double chin as well.

Cheek muscles can be toned by blowing both cheeks out while holding your mouth closed, then by sucking both cheeks inwardly so your lips are protruding out like a fish.

II. NECK

Neck muscles are often neglected in considering exercises. The three main groups of muscles to consider are the ones that turn your head right and left; the ones that bend your head forward to the chin-on-chest position and back to chin-turned-up position; and the ones that bend your head to the ear-on-the-shoulder positions.

The easiest way to exercise neck muscles is to position your head and neck in any of the six positions mentioned, then force your neck in the opposite direction against the resistance of your hand. For example, with your head turned to the left, turn it to the right against the resistance of your right hand lying alongside your right forehead. Bend your neck backward from the chin-on-chest position against the resistance of your hands clasped alongside the back of your head. Bend your neck from the left ear-on-shoulder position against the resistance of your right hand lying alongside your right temple. You can increase or decrease the pressure of the resisting hand. Since these muscles are seldom used, it's wise to take it easy at first—don't force too hard. Expect to hear some "creaking" of neck ligaments with these exercises—it's quite safe.

III. SHOULDERS

You can strengthen your shoulders in a number of ways. A simple isometric method is to elevate one shoulder against the resistance of the opposite hand pulling downward on it. Another way is to lean against a door frame with only your shoulder supporting your weight against it. Suddenly, make your shoulder forcefully push your body away from the frame. Reverse this by turning around and leaning against the frame with the back part of your shoulder and push away by suddenly forcing your shoulder backward.

Using a small weight is another good way to strengthen shoulders. Using a ten pound bell—the short bar that comes with weight sets with a five pound weight at either end—slowly elevate the weight from alongside your leg to a point where your arm is extended straight above your head, then back down again. Keep your arm straight at the elbow and make your shoulder muscles do all the lifting. Do this extending your arm forward, sidewise, and to the rear.

Another exercise for your shoulders is to use the long bar of the weight set with twenty to twenty-five pounds on either end. Place the bar on the floor with one weight in the direction you're facing, the other to the rear. Now bend at your knees and waist until you can grab the middle of the bar. Keeping your legs and waist out, make your shoulder muscles pick up the weight until the bar is at the level of your chest, then return the weight to the floor. Repeat this as often as you can, increasing the number of times with time.

If you have a punching bag, boxing the bag, increasing the time you hold your arms up to "punch" will give stamina to your shoulder muscles.

IV. CHEST

One of the bonuses of using weights is that when you grab a weight in almost any position, and lift it or change its position in any way, your shoulder, chest, arm and grip are all helped. The same applies to chinning yourself on one of the basement pipes. Whenever you pull yourself up to the pipe your arms, chest, and grip muscles are benefited.

Your chest muscles can be pulled by simply grasping hands in front of your chest, and pulling in opposite directions with your arms and hands. As you pull, bend your elbows inwardly toward your rib cage to tighten your chest muscles even more. There is nothing like swimming and tennis for chest muscle tone. Hand-ball and chopping wood will also do nicely as variations in toning the chest muscles.

V. ARM

Alternate methods to exercise and tone your arm muscles will help keep the drudgery from your exercise routines. Try extending your arms against any flat wall, using your body as a counterweight against them. Simply make your arms push you away (or pull you toward) the wall or door frame and press your hands against the top of the frame. Usually, you will find that your arms aren't completely extended. Now make your arms straighten out by pushing upward.

Any manipulations of weights while lying flat on the floor is an alternate to standing up and using them. Use the small weights and bar first. When you feel tone returning in your arms, you can switch to the long bar and more weights. Add weights *slowly,* and you'll avoid strain and unnecessary muscle knotting.

Rowing a boat is good arm and chest exercise. Sawing wood will condition arm muscles quite well.

VI. ABDOMEN

One variation to strengthen your abdomen when you've mastered the sit-up in the way I've previously described, is to do sit-ups with a small amout of weight in your hands. Use the small bar and light weights at first. Yet another variation is to do scissor kicks and sit-ups at the same time. This takes a bit of practice, but really keeps that abdomen in shape!

While standing, use a circular motion at your waist muscles—bend forward, to each side, and backwards, hands on hips and using a smooth motion. This keeps the waistline trim. With feet a bit apart, bend to one side as far as possible, arms outstretched, and dipping the arm to the side toward which you bend. Do the same with the opposite side.

Suck in your abdomen until you feel yourself shaking with the exertion, then tighten down your abdominal muscles so that they bend you forward at the waist, hardening your abdominal wall so that you can forcefully dig both thumbs or fists into it without discomfort. This is an alternate isometric for your abdominal muscles.

VII. LEGS

Practice getting up from the floor and standing from a sitting position in a chair without using your arms to help. If you're on the floor, cross both legs, Indian style, then make them hoist you to a standing position without bracing with your arms. This tones up those thigh muscles. While standing, lean against a dresser or door frame with one hand, and reach behind you with the opposite hand to grasp your ankle, bending your knee so you can reach it. Now forcefully straighten your leg against the resistance of your grip on your ankle. This tones up your hamstring muscles—the ones that make the cords in back of your knee joint. Again, swimming, cycling, and just plain walking does wonders for those legs. Enjoy the lift of spirit and feel the exhilaration of a brisk early morning or late evening walk.

C. SALT-FREE AND LOW-SALT DIETS

The function of a low-salt (sometimes called low-sodium) diet is to provide a guide with all the essentials of good nutrition yet low in salt. I've already discussed reasons why this is important to the well-being of your health and good control of low blood sugar.

Some confusion results in using the words "salt" and "sodium" interchangeably. To clarify, sodium is not salt, but salt is made up of nearly half sodium. There are some other products that contain sodium, but not salt—it's the *sodium* you're trying to restrict with so-called low-salt diets.

Remember that baking powder and baking soda also have large quantities of sodium in them. The following formula represents a baking powder that works well, yet has no sodium whatsoever in it. It can be made quite inexpensively at your pharmacist's:

Potassium bicarbonate	39.8 gms.
Cornstarch	28.9 gms.
Tartaric Acid	7.5 gms.
Potassium bitartrate	56.1 gms.

This formula makes about 4½ ounces of good baking powder.

It's also true that in curtailing sodium, you must take into account that many proprietary medicines have a good deal of sodium in them. Among these are some antibiotics, most alkalizers (medicines used for "sour" stomach), cough medicines, laxatives, pain relievers, and sedatives.

In considering your sodium restricted diet, the following food plan will be helpful:

LOW-SALT DIET

Use foods that have been prepared without the addition of salt

RECOMMENDED FOOD PLAN

Meat, Fish or Fowl	Beef	Lamb	Fresh Pork	Tripe
	Chicken	Liver, calves	Rabbit	Veal
	Duck	Liver, pig	Turkey	Oysters
	Beef Heart	Liver, turkey	Tongue, beef	Catfish
	Fresh Salmon	Fresh Halibut	Salt Free Tuna	
Fats	Unsalted butter, Spry, Crisco, unsalted oil salad dressing.			
Cheese	Dry, salt free, cottage cheese, use ⅓ cup as an alternate for 1 cup milk.			
Eggs	One daily.			
Cereals	Cooked cereals (except quick cooking cream of wheat) without added salt, puffed rice, puffed wheat, shredded wheat, and muffets.			
Bread	White, whole wheat or rye, without added salt.			
Potatoes or Alternate	White potatoes, sweet potatoes, rice, spaghetti, macaroni noodles.			
Vegetables	Fresh or frozen vegetables. Also those canned without added salt.			
Fruits	Any fruit (One citrus fruit daily).			
Desserts	Custard, ice cream or pudding if taken from the egg and milk allowance. Fruit juice tapioca. Gelatin desserts made with plain gelatin, fruit and juice.			
Sweets	Those that do not contain added salt or nuts. Sugar, honey, pure jelly and jams, marmalade, and pure sugar candies.			
Milk	Two cups daily.			
Beverages	Coffee, tea, if permitted by physician.			

Foods to Avoid   Table salt, baking powder, soda, spices, celery salt, regular
canned vegetables, frozen peas and lima beans, highly
seasoned food, soup concentrates, smoked fish or meat, ham,
dried beef, canned fish, meats or soups, mayonnaise, all
processed cheese, soda crackers, potato chips, pickles, olives,
pies, cakes and rich desserts, jello, salted nuts, cultured
buttermilk.

SUGGESTED MENU

Breakfast	*Dinner*	*Supper*
Orange, 1	SF Meat, 2½ oz.	SF Meat, 2½ oz.
SF Cereal, ½ cup	SF Buttered Potato, ½ c.	SF Buttered Rice, ½ cup.
SF Egg, 1	SF Buttered Carrots, ½ c.	SF Buttered Green Beans,
SF Toast, 1 slice	SF Bread, 1 slice	½ C.
SF Butter, 1 tsp.	SF Butter, 1 tsp.	SF Bread, 1 slice
Milk, 1 cup	Lettuce Salad with	SF Butter, 1 tsp.
	honey & lemon juice	Canned Peaches, ½ cup.
	dressing	
	Canned Pear, ½ cup.	
	Milk, 1 cup.	

It's also well to remember that water treated in water-softeners is quite
high in sodium.

D. HINTS FOR DIABETICS

Recall that I said that a diabetic diet should be as near to any
other diet as possible with adequate protein and nutrients and no
more calories than needed to gain or reduce to ideal weight.

The only real difference between a diabetic diet and any other is
the relative amounts of carbohydrates and fats. Proteins are essentially
the same. A diabetic should have roughly 50 per cent more fat and
50 per cent fewer carbohydrates than would be usual.

Here are some rules of thumb that you may use to tell how your
diabetic diet should be apportioned:

1. Find your *ideal* weight (from the height-weight-frame tables
   in Chapter 3).
2. At 100 pounds *ideal* weight you need 1400 calories a day if
   you're maintaining your weight. For every ten pounds of ideal
   weight over 100, add 150 calories. This is your daily calorie
   limit.
3. If you're reducing, *subtract* 40 per cent from the calories listed

in Step #2. For example, if you *should* weight 100 pounds and must reduce to get there, your calorie limit is 840 rather than 1400–40 per cent of 1400 = 560. 1400 less 560 = 840.

4. If you're unusually active, add 3 per cent to the total calories as your daily limit from the figure given in #2. For example: If your ideal weight is 100 pounds, and you're unusually active, your daily limit should be increased to 1820 calories— 30 per cent of 1400 equals 420. 1400 + 420 = 1820.

5. 10 per cent of your total daily calorie limit should be taken in carbohydrate: If your daily calorie limit is 1400, then 140 grams of your food should be carbohydrate.

6. Half of this figure should be taken in fat: If you should be taking 140 grams of carbohydrate, then you should have 70 grams of fat every day.

7. Regardless of your calorie limit, you should have 0.5 grams of protein per pound of ideal body weight: If your ideal body weight is 100 pounds, then you should have 50 grams of protein every day.

The following table will show you how much (in grams and calories) some common foods contain:

One ounce serving	Carbohydrate	Protein	Fat	Calories
Bread, one large slice	15	2.5	0	70
Oatmeal, large portion	20	5	2	118
Crackers, four squares	20	3	2	110
* Vegetables	1	0.3	0	5
Potato	6	1	0	28
Milk	1.5	1	1	19
Egg, one	0	6	6	78
Meat, lean	0	7	5	73
Chicken, lean	0	8	3	59
Fish, fat-free	0	6	0	24
Cheese	0	8	10	122
Bacon	0	5	15	155
Cream, light	1	1	6	62
Cream, heavy	1	1	12	116
Butter	0	0	25	225

* The following vegetables contain *twice* the values listed in this table:

Tomatoes	Onions	Green Peas
Turnips	Squash	Pumpkin
Carrots	Brussels Sprouts	
Okra	Beets	

For convenience, remember that 30 grams equal one ounce.

Remember that proper *weight and diet* often control adult diabetes without other treatment. Exercise makes such control *even more efficient.* One of the oral diabetic drugs can be added if diet and exercise are not enough. If this proves not effective, insulin can be started.

Index